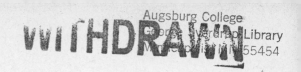
Take Charge

A Strategic
Guide for
Blind Job Seekers

Rabby & Croft

National Braille Press Inc.
Boston, Massachusetts

Excerpts from Joyce Lain Kennedy's career columns were reprinted through the courtesy of Sun Features Inc., © 1988. Joyce Lain Kennedy is the author of the nationally syndicated newspaper feature CAREERS.

Excerpts from "A Shortage of Youths Brings Wide Changes to the Labor Market" reprinted by permission of *The Wall Street Journal*, © Dow Jones & Company, Inc., September 2, 1986. All Rights Reserved.

Excerpt from "Some Advice to Blind Interviewers" reprinted by permission of *The Braille Monitor*, © National Federation of the Blind, Inc., June-July 1987. All Rights Reserved.

"Male Executives Also Suffer for Their Sartorial Mistakes" reprinted by permission of *The Wall Street Journal*, © Dow Jones & Company, Inc., September 1, 1987. All Rights Reserved.

"Businesswomen's Broader Latitude in Dress Codes Goes Just So Far" reprinted by permission of *The Wall Street Journal*, © Dow Jones & Company, Inc., September 1, 1987. All Rights Reserved.

Excerpts from CAREERSEARCH reprinted by permission of The Erdlen Bograd Group, Inc., Wellesley, Mass.

ISBN: 0-939173-16-6

PRINTED IN THE UNITED STATES OF AMERICA

Dedication

This book is dedicated to the "salmon"
who have been swimming upstream for generations,
with scars on their bellies to prove it.

This book is for you . . .

. . . the unemployed, but determined-to-be-employed, blind job seeker.

. . . the employed, but determined-to-be-*better*-employed, blind job seeker.

. . . the savvy parent of a blind child, who sees a brighter future.

. . . the smart rehabilitation counselor who understands who's in charge.

. . . the conscientious teacher who provides career counseling.

. . . the employer who wants to be prepared for the next take-charge blind job seeker who walks through the door.

§

Table of Contents

Preface

The employment picture for disabled job seekers has never looked better. Four forces are coming together right now to create a more favorable environment: changing employer needs, changing employer attitudes, the rapid pace of technological development, and the attitudes of blind people themselves.

We are moving from a "baby boom" generation, wherein employers had their pick of employees, to a "baby bust" generation, such that employers will be scrambling for workers. Many of the new entrants into the work force by the year 2000 will be people who traditionally have been disadvantaged.

At the same time, the social changes of the '60s and early '70s have paved the way for enlightened attitudes toward the integration of people with "differences." Already, the work force in this country has changed dramatically from a predominately white, able-bodied male majority to a work force which includes women, minorities, and people with disabilities. *By the year 2000, 80% of all new entrants into the American work force will be women, minorities, or immigrants.*

Advances in technology will continue to improve the work lives of people with disabilities, reducing the impact of the disability on job performance and productivity. No crystal ball can foretell the incredible influence these developments will have on all our lives.

Concurrently, we who are blind are moving to integrate ourselves, on an equal footing, into the general labor market—asserting our right to be part of the diverse working world. We see ourselves as part of, rather than separate from, society at large. This book not only reflects this trend, but unabashedly encourages and celebrates it.

The times, they are a'changing.

With change come new ways of looking at situations. Until very recently, we who were blind and looking for work relied on rehabilitation counselors to identify, search for, and locate suitable jobs for us. It's time for us to assume personal responsibility for our own job-search campaigns—and the outcome. It's time for us to take charge of our own career explorations, making use of the same resources and services available to sighted career changers, job seekers, and workers.

This book will help you think about, and make independent decisions about, strategies which meet your unique needs. **Take Charge** is a practical self-help guide built upon the real-life experiences of blind people. Most of the strategies recommended in this book have been proved successful by at least some blind job seekers. In fact, for the purpose of this book, we organized a day-long seminar on employment strategies, which was attended by successfully employed blind individuals. Their comments are peppered throughout the book.

This book addresses the current status of employment opportunities for people who are blind. It recognizes that we have not reached the ideal, when our blindness will be no more important than the color of our hair. It proposes strategies for dealing with a resistant labor market. This book aims to assist blind readers in unraveling the complexities of the labor market and of life in the workplace; analyzing jobs; focusing on one's true career interests and work-related skills; networking one's way to the personal attention of a hiring manager; probing an interviewer's state of mind and conclusions about one's candidacy; and strategizing one's way out of frustrating work situations.

There will be many times, as you ponder your employment future, when you will feel discouraged. Remember that the employment picture for people with disabilities is moving forward every day. History proves that public attitudes of the majority toward the minority move along a continuum, from fear and hostility to acceptance. We who are blind have not reached the end of the spectrum. We will. Movement will come as we take individual actions which, collectively, cause a lurch forward along this continuum toward acceptance.

Thirty-four years ago, Rosa Parks, a black woman, refused to give up her seat on a bus to a white woman. Her singular action prompted a collective impatience now known as the civil rights movement. It is hard to comprehend that 34 years ago, Rosa Parks not only had to stand when a white person wanted a seat on the bus; she also had to pay her fare in the front of the bus and then get off, walk to the back, and enter through the rear door. Today no one would accept this standard.

Today an employer may believe it's okay to ask a blind job applicant how he or she will get to work. Tomorrow no one will accept this standard.

The action you take today will affect that tomorrow.

§

A Look Ahead

Just for fun, let's take a peek at the other end of the spectrum.

* * * *

6:00 a.m. The year is 2010. A soft-spoken female voice says, "Wake up, Jim. Today is the best day of your life." The international marketing manager for a major network conglomerate, awakened by his talking-computer alarm, listens for the preprogrammed weather report for Moscow, where he will be spending the next few days negotiating a network deal. "Sunny and clear."

Meet Jim Bolt, a manager of the future who happens to be blind.

Our fictitious character doesn't think much about his blindness, though. Juggling a hectic work load—darting from country to country—consumes most of his energy. The rest he devotes to his wife and nine-year-old daughter, Symbella.

Jim ambles out of bed and touches a button on his speech-activated computer: "Jim, your tickler file says, 'It's time to have your teeth re-pearled, and don't forget about Symbella's birthday next week.' Today's schedule is: eight thirty a.m. meeting with . . . ."

7:00 a.m. Jim checks his pocket for his credit-card-size reading machine and EZMoneyCard, grabs his intelligent navigational aid, and heads out for the supertram. His suitcase was picked up the night before by Magic Carpet Express, guaranteeing delivery in Moscow upon his arrival. He leaves instructions on his personal computer for it to call Krazy Kat Klothes and charge his account for a gift for Symbella, as well as the Gourmet Tele-Cake to order his daughter's favorite flavor—double chocolate chip crunch—with the appropriate number of candles.

He stops by Fast Break, grabs a grab-and-eat breakfast package, pops it into the store microwave to heat it, pays for it, and continues on his way.

On the tram, there is just enough time for Jim to check his electronic mailbox and to read the sports section of the *Washington Satellite Times* via his portable braille laptop. The Redskins lost. He keys in a reminder to pay a lost wager to Dave in Accounting.

7:50 a.m. Jim arrives at his high-tech office, where an electronically-timed, freshly brewed cup of organic coffee awaits him. He calls his executive assistant in to go over some last-minute details for his trip. The assistant reminds Jim that he has a salary review at 8:30, via video screen, with his boss, who is working in Spain. Jim asks his assistant to locate the laser card that contains his most recent sales figures, in preparation for a tough negotiation. The executive assistant reminds Jim that *his* review is two weeks overdue, and Jim agrees to handle his assistant's review immediately after his own. With administrative personnel in short supply, Jim knows he must reward his assistant with a bonus, in addition to his annual increase.

10:00 a.m. At a staff meeting, Jim finds himself in the middle of a power struggle between two division heads which threatens to undermine an important network deal with an Asian producer. He quickly intervenes, makes them aware of the stakes, and works out a compromise. He agrees to reconsider his own position regarding one of the contract specifications.

11:30 a.m. Jim presses a preprogrammed button on his wireless phone, which alerts the cab company that he needs a ride to the airport. Once there, Jim slips his EZMoneyCard into a machine which prints out his ticket, and he steps onto a moveable sidewalk which drops him at the right gate.

12:45 p.m. The SuperConcorde lifts off, and Jim reaches for the headphones to listen to a tape on conversational Russian, his third language. A few minutes into the lesson, Jim finds himself daydreaming about ways to spend the new compensation package he negotiated for himself that morning. His fantasy takes him to a remote island teeming with rainbow trout, far from the sounds of electronic machines that have come to dominate his life.

Abruptly, his pleasant thoughts are crowded out by a memory of the fishing trip he never made. He was 10 years old, a Boy Scout, and ready for adventure. The troop had planned an all-day deep-sea fishing excursion. It would be his first. But someone objected; he never knew who. How could a blind boy fish? What if he fell overboard? Who would bait his line? Wouldn't he ruin the trip for the others?

Jim smiled. How things had changed. No one would dream of making such stupid comments today. Everybody knows that you don't need to see to fish, or to do much else for that matter. Most of the inconveniences of blindness have been reduced by training and technology—the rest calls for a little *chutzpah*.

Jim picks up the videophone located near his seat and dials home. He wants to tell his wife about his raise, and to let Symbella know that he'll be there for her birthday. Thank goodness for the SuperConcorde. How did people manage in the past?

§

Acknowledgments

Funding from the following organizations made this book possible—and affordable:

American Brotherhood for the Blind
The Boston Globe Foundation II, Inc.
Digital Equipment Corporation
National Federation of the Blind
New England Telephone
Raytheon Company

We wanted this book to be steeped in reality, so we asked a group of successfully employed blind individuals to meet with us for a day to discuss employment strategies. Their comments anchor this book. We wish to thank:

Steven Booth
Sharlene Czaja
Judith Dixon
Olga Espinola
Al Gayzagian
Marie Hennessy
Bill Raeder

Barry Scheur
Peter Slowkowski
Rosemary Teehan
David Ticchi
Jeff Turner
Gayle Yarnall
Duncan Watson

Ed Colozzi, a career/life counselor in Hawaii, spent considerable time modifying his career-exploration workbook to accompany this book. We appreciate his wise counsel.

To check our thinking, we asked five people to bring their intellects to bear on the manuscript. It was an enormous assignment which they tackled with fervor. As happens, not all reviewers agreed with all of the strategies presented in this book, but most of their comments are reflected in the final product. We are indebted to:

Judith M. Dixon, Ph.D., head, Consumer Relations Section, National Library Service for the Blind and Physically Handicapped of the Library of Congress

John D. Erdlen, president, The Erdlen Bograd Group, Inc., a human-resources consulting firm

Al Gayzagian, financial officer, John Hancock Insurance Company

James S. Nyman, Ph.D., director of Services for the Visually Impaired, State of Nebraska, Department of Public Institutions

Barry Scheur, private attorney, Scheur Management

The process of publishing a book might be described as revise, revise, revise. Several people at National Braille Press deserve recognition:

Phyllis Campana, who trimmed the fat
Joan Hanson, who tenderized the meat
Paul Griffitts, who prepared the cuisine

Credit for the audio edition goes to:
Carl de Suze, who turned the prose into music
Ray Fournier, who orchestrated the concert
Chris Engles, who edited the sound track
Jim Michaels, who confiscated the outtakes

Finally, we wish to thank the employers who agreed to be interviewed for this book. ¤

Chapter 1
Exploring the Possibilities

Most of us would rank near the bottom if quizzed on that ubiquitous subject, *work*. We spend 12-20 years studying everything from algebra to zoology, but we neglect probably the highest-payback subject of all: the study of work.

The problem dates back to our otherwise prophetic forefathers, who settled for reading, writing, and arithmetic when the world was a simpler place. Work didn't need to be studied, it needed to be done.

What a difference a bicentennial makes.

In today's world, work is a big subject. The U.S. Bureau of Labor Statistics reports there are 20,000 job categories in the world of work today. *That translates into 20,000 job possibilities for you to consider.*

Tomorrow, there will be more. Chances are, you only know about a handful of these. And if you're blind and looking for work, there's a good possibility that you have further limited your job options based on "what a blind person could do."

Not to worry. To get the right job for you, you don't need to study 20,000 jobs; what you do need to do is expand your horizons a bit. And, you need to study work.

Otherwise, you will have a tendency—like so many of us do—to look at jobs superficially. Dan Rather makes journalism look intriguing, until you read that journalism is ranked *the sixth most stressful occupation in the work force,* after miner, police officer, pilot, prison guard, and construction worker.

Looking at jobs without careful scrutiny leads to false assumptions which can have a serious effect on your search for the right job. You may suppose that few jobs are more tedious than that of a postal worker, following a mindless routine in inclement weather. What you fail to consider are the *intangible* aspects of the job, as described by this thirty-year postal veteran:

"I love every minute of it. I'm part of the community, like a cop on a beat. I know every kid on the block by name. I give them a push on their bikes, or throw back a Frisbee . . . they wait for me every day.

"And there's a comradeship in the mailroom, a lot of joking around. People care about each other. Plus, you know, no matter what's happening in the economy, you can support your family."

These "hidden" aspects of a job—environment, peers, purpose, status, job security, autonomy—can make or break a job, depending on who you are. To protect yourself from a lifetime of unhappiness in the work force, you need to uncover both the tangible and intangible aspects of any job, and study their effect on you. Studying work is hard work. But it's worth it.

You can't afford not to.

IGNORANCE IS YOUR BIGGEST HANDICAP

You can't afford (we're talking dollars and sense here) to remain ignorant about the world of work. Not if you want to be part of it, because:

1. Ignorance limits your career options.
2. Ignorance reduces your chances of getting a job.
3. Ignorance ultimately affects your job satisfaction.
4. Ignorance keeps you from developing a philosophy about how you, as a blind person, will compete.

2

1. Ignorance Limits
Your Career Options

Ask a child, "What do you want to be when you grow up?" and you're likely to get: "nurse," "wrestler," "fireman," "mommy." Why not. Kids, for the most part, learn about the world of work from what they see on TV or from watching what their parents do. Unless their parents do it, they don't think about becoming a certified public accountant with a small investment firm, a make-up artist with a major movie studio, or an anesthesiologist.

The educational system in this country provides us with the technical knowledge of psychology, computers, or the arts, but not with the personal knowledge of how these fields of interest might sustain us in a rewarding career.

Consequently, many of us will spend the rest of our lives in search of satisfying work, not knowing what would make us happy because we lack the knowledge and wisdom about work that we thought could only come from direct experience.

It doesn't have to be that way. We could come out of school with a much better idea of what we really want to do. And, today, kids who get good career counseling do. *It is entirely possible, with some determination and a lot of study, to discover what you want to do and how to get a job doing it.*

You *can* improve your chances of selecting a career that matches your skills, values, and sense of excitement *before* you are too old, too broke, or too tired to go back to school and start all over.

The first step is to e-x-p-a-n-d your thinking about the jobs you could potentially do. As a blind person, you may have limited your options based on what your parents or rehabilitation counselor think is possible, or based on what jobs are "good for a blind person."

Another myth shattered.

No one knows how many different types of jobs are being performed by blind people. No sooner have we concluded that a particular job cannot be performed without sight than we hear about a blind person who is doing exactly that job. Consider this *partial* listing, compiled by Job Opportunities for the Blind (JOB), a joint project of the Department of Labor and the National Federation of the Blind, in Baltimore, Maryland, of jobs being performed by blind employees. Of course, this does not represent all of the types of jobs blind people are doing; it is merely a sampling:

Administrative Assistant
Administrative Technician
Administrator
Advocacy Coordinator
Airline Reservationist
Assembler, Electronics
Assembler, General
Assembly Line Worker, Airline Factory
Assistant Attorney General
Assistant Director, College Alumni Assoc.
Assistant Professor of Psychology
Banker, Senior Vice President
Cane Travel Instructor
Chaplain
Child Care Worker
Client Assistance Project Worker
Collections Officer
Computer Operator
Computer Programmer
Computer Systems Analyst
Cosmetologist
Counselor, Adolescent
Counselor, Business Enterprise Program
Counselor, College
Counselor, Housing Complaints
Counselor, Rehabilitation

Custodian
Customer Service Representative
Darkroom Technician
Disabled Student Advisor
Dispatcher
Dog Groomer
Economist
Employment Development Specialist
Engineer, Electrical
Engineer, Safety
Equal Opportunity Employment Officer
Estate Analyst
Farmer
File Clerk
Film Processor
Fixed Income Portfolio Analyst
Fund Raiser
Gas Station Attendant
Greenhouse Worker
Handicapped Service Coordinator
Health Club Manager
Homemaker Aide
Hotline Coordinator
Independent Living Skills Coordinator
Information Clerk/Specialist
Inside Sales Vice President, Publishing
Insurance Sales Representative
Intake Social Worker
International Marketing Manager
Internal Revenue Service Financial Assistant
Internal Revenue Service Tax Examiner
Internal Revenue Service Taxpayer Service Representative
Investment Manager
Janitor
Job Development Specialist
Journalist
Judge

Labor Relations Specialist
Lawyer
Legislator
Librarian
Loan Coordinator
Machinist
Mail Clerk
Maintenance Mechanic
Management Consultant
Marketing Representative
Masseur/Masseuse
Mathematician
Mechanic, Automotive
Mental Health Counselor
Meteorologist
Micrographic Technician
Minister
National Park Service Employee
Newspaper Bundler
Nurse's Aide
Nutrition Education Coordinator
Occupational Health and Safety Specialist
Occupational Therapist
Office Supply Store Employee
Operations Clerk
Order Taker
Packager and Loader
Parole Officer
PBX Operator
Personnel Interviewer
Personnel Specialist
Pharmacist
Photo Finish Worker
Physical Therapist
Placement Specialist
Principal
Professor

Propagation Manager
Psychiatrist, Psychologist
Public School Visual Impairments Specialist
Quality Control Specialist
Radio Announcer/Producer
Radio and TV Repairer
Radio Reading Services, Assistant Manager
Realtor
Receptionist
Recreational Therapist
Reference Librarian, Adult Services
Rehabilitation Teacher
Research Analyst
Restaurant Worker
Router at Bank
Sales Executive
Salesperson, Retail
Salesperson, Telephone
Secretary
Security Guard
Senior Processor
Shipping/Receiving Clerk
Small Business Owner
Social Worker
Speech Pathologist
Staff Assistant Supervisor
Stockbroker
Store Manager
Strategic Planner
Systems Planner, Hospital
Switchboard Operator
Talent Agent
Teacher and Teacher's Aide
Telemarketing Representative
Tour Guide
Trade Specialist
Transcriber, Medical

Translator
Travel Agent
Typist, Dictaphone
Typist, Mag Card II
Typist, Receptionist
Typist, Word Processing
University Instructor
Volunteer Coordinator/Computer Skills
Volunteer Coordinator/Fund Raiser
Woodworker

Once you open your mind to the full range of career options available to you, you need to expand your thinking even further. Selecting a field of interest is just part of the equation; next you need to explore all of the possibilities *within* that field.

Take the insurance field, for example. Career consultant Joyce Lain Kennedy has written in her career column, "There's much more than meets the eye in the insurance business, such as accountants, appraisers, arson investigators, attorneys, business managers, chemists, computer programmers, editors, fire protection engineers, industrial hygienists, librarians, public relations specialists, make up the gigantic insurance industry of nearly 2 million people."

Even after you have narrowed down your job options, you need to think of the many different environments in which you could practice your occupation. Nursing is a good example of this. You could be a nurse in the Peace Corps, in the military, in the State Department, at a school, in a nursing home, in a health care maintenance organization (HMO), in the emergency room, in the operating room, for an insurance company, for a hospice, or at the publishing office of *American Nurse*.

Each one of these choices will affect your job satisfaction. You may thrive on being a nurse in the emergency room, but not at a hospice or nursing home.

2. Ignorance Reduces Your Chances of Getting a Job

Tell a personnel manager that you want a job in personnel "because you like people," and she will probably smile and escort you to the door.

She knows (and you should know) that people in personnel handle wage and salary administration, pensions, and benefits. They prepare manuals on training or company policies; collect statistics and do job analyses; comply with state and federal regulations; maintain files and issue forms. And, worst of all, people in personnel spend a great deal of time *rejecting* people. Since only one person will get the job, the others have to be told—by you—that they didn't.

Or maybe you've been thinking about a career in public relations, where you could use your well-developed social skills? In truth, effective public relations depends on good *graphics* and good *writing*, as well as good contacts.

Back to the drawing board.

The point is, unless you know a good deal about the job you are applying for, you probably won't get past the first interview. Few things are more annoying to a hiring manager than wasting time with a candidate who isn't adequately informed about the job at hand.

Here's how a senior department head for a large computer division explained her reaction to a blind job seeker who applied for a computer programmer position and who hadn't done his homework:

"This fellow had written one simple program for the PC and decided he wanted to be a computer programmer. The local rehabilitation agency referred him to us. I asked him, 'What do you think you'll be doing every day?' He said, 'Writing programs.' I responded, 'Most of the time you won't be writing programs.' He didn't have a clue about the job, and I wasn't impressed."

A senior manager in a large insurance company (who himself is blind) describes a similar experience with a blind applicant:

"A young man came in to apply for a job as an underwriter. I asked him how he planned to do the job. He replied, 'With my Optacon.' Of course, most of the work is handwritten, and the Optacon can't read handwriting. So, although this particular job isn't one that a totally blind person can perform—at least not with the technology currently available—he reduced his chances of getting any job with the company by demonstrating his lack of preparation."

3. Ignorance Ultimately Affects Your Job Satisfaction

You probably know a teacher who doesn't want to be a teacher, a nurse who hates nursing, a lawyer who wishes she had gone into another profession.

On the surface, the jobs looked good. The teacher envisioned a job that ended at 3:30, with summers off, only to discover that it also requires 2-3 hours every night to grade papers and prepare lesson plans. The flight attendant dreamed of exotic travel, but finds herself too weary after 13-hour shifts of smiling and serving—and fending off unwanted attentions. The advertising executive wants to create, but finds that his clients have their own ideas, and soon his work becomes just another ad. The telephone operator wants to talk to people, but the company rule is "no talking to customers."

The sad part is, all of this information was readily available to these professionals *before* they fell victim to their jobs. They chose their lots too hastily, without conducting the necessary investigation into their occupations.

You don't have to make that mistake.

All jobs are part of a larger system. They exist within a certain environment (corporate, human service, private, public), they coexist within a peer group (white collar, blue collar, pink collar), they involve a time commitment (from minimal to every waking hour), they come with a relative status (which varies from one culture to another, from one decade to the next), and they come with other "extras" (autonomy, isolation, chaos, variety, and so on).

The smart job seeker knows that these intangible aspects of any given job often have a greater impact on job satisfaction than the actual job tasks do.

4. Ignorance Keeps You from Developing a Philosophy About How You, As a Blind Person, Will Compete

Employers want to hire problem solvers, not problems. Which means that *you*, not the employer, have to be prepared to think through your own job problems and devise solutions for them. The more you know about the world of work, the better able you will be to figure out what alternative techniques you should use, what being "productive" means, and what interpersonal style you should adopt. Designing strategies for yourself in a work setting is an evolutionary process that involves both knowledge and experience.

But before you tackle a prospective employer's expectations of you, you need to have some of your own. How will you measure your own productivity, compared to others'? Do you expect to compete equally with your sighted peers? What does that mean? Can you do so even if you want to? How will you know if you do?

All of these nagging questions evolve into a philosophy that will affect your performance on the job, and the eventual outcome of your career. A philosophy which will, no doubt, change as you gain experience in working side by side with other workers. Attitude and approach are two big words in the world of work. Both require careful thinking.

KNOW WHERE YOU'RE GOING

It all adds up to the same thing: The more you know about work and the more you know about yourself, the better your chances are of finding something that you will enjoy waking up to each morning. What you don't know will work against you.

Count on it.

The real secret behind job satisfaction is knowing who you are, what you need (enjoy), what you value, and what jobs exist to meet those needs. The next section presents four strategies for learning more about the world of work, and improving your chances of getting the right job for you.

FOUR STRATEGIES FOR
LEARNING MORE ABOUT WORK

Here are four ways to begin your course of study about the world of work:

1. Reading,
2. Asking and Listening,
3. Observing, and
4. Actually Working.

Strategy No. 1: Reading

The amount of reading material for the job hunter is truly overwhelming. In *print*, that is. As you know, only a minuscule amount of this information is available in braille, large print, or recorded form. It only makes sense, therefore, to avail yourself of everything that is accessible, and to find competent readers to handle the rest.

1. Send for a cassette called "A Job in Your Future," free, from *Dialogue* magazine. And for a three-cassette pack called "The Assertive Job Seeker" (price: $12.00) from In-Touch Networks. Also, you can order a cassette called "Marketing Your Abilities" (price: $3.95) from Mainstream Inc. All three publications are filled with helpful advice for the blind and otherwise disabled job hunter.

2. Subscribe to direct-circulation magazines in your occupational field produced by the National Library Service for the Blind and Physically Handicapped (NLS), such as: *Fortune* (braille), *Foreign Affairs* (talking book), *Journal of Counselling and Development* (talking book), *Psychology Today* (braille), *Social Work* (talking book), *Personal Computing* (braille), *Horizon* (braille), *Journal of Rehabilitation* (braille), *Farm Journal* (talking book), *Popular Mechanics* (braille), *Writer* (talking book), *National Geographic* (talking book), etc. Subscriptions are free from your regional library for the blind and physically handicapped.

In addition to the magazines in the direct-circulation program, there are other magazines, produced by volunteers on cassette, such as *Forbes* and *Barron's*, which may be available through your regional library.

Other organizations sell subscriptions for a wide variety of occupationally-oriented publications. Recorded Periodicals of Philadelphia, Pennsylvania, for example, makes available *Broadcasting*, *Radio Digest*, *ComputerWorld*, *Scientific American*, and *Science News*, among others. All of them are on cassette, for varying prices, depending on whether you borrow them or keep them. Send for a complete listing.

3. While you're talking to your regional library, order the NLS reference circular called "From School to Working Life: Resources and Services." Also, remember that you can order from your regional library (or directly from NLS) comprehensive bibliographies on any subject—including

career planning, job hunting, and employment. The books listed are all available in accessible media. Simply specify the subject area.

4. Send for a list of free publications available from the JOB Project in Baltimore, Maryland. It includes, among other things, recordings of JOB-sponsored seminars, articles, pamphlets, and the regular JOB Applicant Bulletin on cassette. Incidentally, JOB Applicant Bulletin No. 106 includes a bibliography of NLS-produced books on careers and employment.

5. Order a cassette called "The Working Blind" (price: $12.00) from National Public Radio. It contains interviews with successfully employed blind people.

6. Get a subscription to *Dialogue* (price: $20.00 for four quarterly issues) and for *Lifeprints*, a magazine for blind young adults (price: $15.00 for five issues a year) from Blindskills, Inc. Both contain regular columns on careers and are available in braille, large print, and recorded formats.

7. Subscribe to the *Harvard Business Review* on cassette (price: $8.50 per bimonthly issue) from the Massachusetts Association for the Blind, and to the Newstrack Executive Tape Service (price: $199 for 24 issues a year) from Newstrack. The Newstrack cassettes contain selected recordings from a variety of business magazines.

8. Send for *Careers and the Handicapped* (price: $5.00 per semiannual issue) from Equal Opportunity Publications. Although this publication is in print, it contains a center section in braille which includes an overview of some of the articles, as well as a list of the advertisers—help wanted advertisers, that is.

9. Send for a list of publications from the President's Committee on Employment of People With Disabilities in Washington, DC, and subscribe, at no cost, to *Worklife*, which the Committee plans to produce on cassette.

10. Finish this book.

These are ten things you can do right now, but the search for work—rewarding, satisfying work—is a much longer process involving a continuous (throughout your lifetime) search for information. Finding work is a full-time job. If you're spending 10 or 20 hours a week on the process, you're going to come up short. The successful job hunter is the one who spends 40 hours a week tracking every lead, and leaving no stone unturned.

Since you clearly are one of those smart job hunters, here are eight places to look for information about the world of work:

I. Public Libraries

Public libraries contain perhaps the best and most comprehensive collection of labor market reading materials. A well-stocked public library will have on its shelves employment-related dictionaries, encyclopedias, and other reference works; government reports and analyses; career and job-hunting books; specialized employment magazines; and newspapers (both local and out-of-town) which carry job vacancy advertisements as well as regular columns on employment.

Great, you say, *but they're all in print*. True, but don't let that stop you. There are several strategies for accessing the abundant job-seeking information sitting on the shelves of your local library.

First, as a long-term strategy, you might take advantage of the corps of volunteers most libraries recruit. As one librarian said, "I don't think there's a library in the country that doesn't have volunteers." If you want to pursue this strategy, here is what several librarians suggested you do:

(a) Call ahead and explain your situation ("I'm blind and looking for work. I need to reference some career books in your library.") Don't just walk in and expect someone to help you;

(b) Help the librarian explore possibilities, *e.g.*, Does the library have a Kurzweil reading machine, a large-print monitor, or facilities for recording? Could the library recruit a volunteer(s) to donate some reading time to this project? Give the library plenty of advance notice. It takes time to mobilize volunteers;

(c) In exchange, offer to volunteer some of your time to the library, answering the phone, babysitting kids while their parents look for books, setting up a story hour, etc. (This is a great way to discover what goes on inside a library);

(d) Never assume that the library owes you this courtesy, but many librarians said they would do everything possible to help make their library collections accessible. Several of the larger ones are planning to purchase equipment to make print materials accessible to blind and visually impaired patrons.

If you feel uncertain about this approach, consider the experiences of these blind patrons who participated in the employment seminar:

"You don't have to present yourself as a 'problem' to the local library. Call ahead and find out what resources they have.

"Some years ago, when I was in law school, I had difficulty using the law library. I called up the head of the library and arranged a meeting to discuss the problem. I found out that the university had a Kurzweil reading machine sitting in the nursing school, collecting dust. I said to the library director, 'Let's work together on this. I'll call Kurzweil and get someone over here to set up and repair the machine. You call the nursing school and get the machine moved over here.' That's exactly what we did.

"Another strategy I would have suggested, if we couldn't get the machine moved to the law library, would have been to have my reader borrow the materials from the library, photocopy them, and return them the same day."

Here is another perspective from a blind employee at a library:

"A good librarian is worth his or her weight in gold. I once asked a reference librarian what her job was. She said, 'My job is to help you focus on what you need. If you're looking at careers, I can tell you where we keep them, under what section, and what's where. In other words, if you come in with a specific problem, we try to get the right resources to you . . . .

"'The biggest problem is people who don't really know what they're looking for; we have to keep asking them questions, instead of vice versa. I have to ask, "Is this what you're looking for?" Sometimes, it takes me an hour just to figure out what they want.'

"So it's not as if sighted people don't walk into the library and ask for assistance—sometimes a lot of assistance. While our situation has some differences, I don't think we should see ourselves as the only people needing help."

On the other hand, if you need to access library materials at a moment's notice, which you will in your job search campaign, there is no substitute for recruiting your own army of readers and having them available to you at your convenience, rather than relying on the availability of the library's volunteers. (We will discuss the recruitment and use of good readers later in this book.)

By the way, in the Fall 1980 issue of *The Occupational Outlook Quarterly*, there is an excellent article entitled "The Job Hunter's Guide to the Library." It was recorded in JOB's Applicant Bulletin No. 61.

II. Specialized Libraries

Some towns have specialized libraries devoted to particular subjects, fields of study, professions, industries, or parts of the world. Such libraries are often located at corporate headquarters, graduate and professional schools (including the career placement and guidance office), trade and professional associations, even at the embassies or consulates of foreign countries. Citibank, for example, has a major library devoted to banking, finance, investment, and economics in New York City. The American Management Association, also in New York City, not only houses an outstanding library on all management subjects, but also offers an excellent information service which is available by phone to its members.

III. The Government

Both the federal and state governments publish enormous amounts of statistical and narrative literature—more, in fact, than you could possibly want to read. An excellent source of information is *The Occupational Outlook Quarterly*, published by the U.S. Department of Labor and replete with articles of interest to the labor market novice.

You may also contact the office of the superintendent of documents of the U.S. Government Printing Office at its Washington, DC, headquarters or at its 15 or so regional branches, and ask for a free bibliography of government publications entitled "Careers and Employment." The U.S. Bureau of Labor Statistics (BLS) conducts and publishes the results of many wage and salary surveys, another area you should study before you begin your job search.

Two publications considered to be the "bibles" of every labor market novice are the *Dictionary of Occupational Titles* and the *Occupational Outlook Handbook*. You can purchase these publications from the BLS Chicago sales office, or study them at any of BLS's nine regional offices. Many of the career-related publications of the U.S. Department of Labor (some of which are now out of print) have been recorded by the JOB Project.

IV. Publishers of Books and Software

A number of publishing houses specialize in career books and literature, such as Ten Speed Press of Berkeley, California, publisher of such giants as *What Color Is Your Parachute?*, *The Three Boxes of Life*, *Where Do I Go From Here With My Life?*, *Don't Use A Resume*, and *Who's Hiring Who*.

Chronicle Guidance Publications of Moravia, New York, offers a particularly good series of regularly updated four-page occupational briefs which describe particular occupations, the tasks involved, the required qualifications, and related trade and professional associations.

If you don't have the patience to seek out these specialist houses, you may prefer to get on the mailing lists of distributors of employment-related literature. Two such distributors are the New Careers Center of Boulder, Colorado, producer of the *Whole Work Catalog*, and JIST Works of Indianapolis, Indiana.

Some computer software publishers are also specializing in career-related software, such as Cambridge Career Products of Charleston, West Virginia.

V. Newsletters and Magazines

As the labor force becomes more diverse, and as jobs become more specialized, magazines and newsletters crop up to meet the new demand.

There are countless examples of this, like *Minority Engineer*, *Working Woman*, *Career World*, a magazine for high school students, and *Collegiate Career Woman*, targeted at college-age and recently graduated females.

A weekly publication aimed at middle- and senior-level managers is *The National Business Employment Weekly*, which is published every Sunday by Dow Jones and Company. And for people looking for a job in the federal government, there's the *Federal Jobs Digest*. As we mentioned before, there is even a career-related magazine targeted to people with disabilities called *Careers and the Handicapped*, which contains job ads directed to disabled job applicants.

Some magazines, while not devoted exclusively to employment issues, run columns or sections on the subject. Three examples are *Changing Times*, *Money*, and *Forbes*; the first two are direct circulation magazines produced on talking book discs by NLS and available from your regional library, while the third is recorded on cassette by volunteers and may be available from your regional library.

There are newsletters for teachers, newsletters for accountants, newsletters for farmers, newsletters for funeral directors, newsletters for small-business owners—well, you get the point. There's a publication out there for you.

VI. Newspapers
Most major newspapers run career-related columns. One of the best known of these is written by Joyce Lain Kennedy, who appears in several hundred newspapers nationwide. (Many of her columns are regularly recorded by the JOB Project in the JOB Applicant Bulletin.) Another is "The Labor Letter," which appears in the Tuesday edition of *The Wall Street Journal*.

Both *The New York Times* and *The Washington Post* publish annual or semiannual supplements on employment trends, the impact of technology on the work force, and education and retraining programs for a changing work world. If these newspapers aren't available in your local library, check a nearby college or university library.

VII. Self-Help Tapes
The market is exploding with motivational, instructional, and employment-related tapes, which can be found in bookstores

and public libraries. Some good sources for such tapes are Career Track in Boulder, Colorado, the Fred Pryor Resource Center in Shawnee Mission, Kansas, and the Nightingale-Conant Corporation in Chicago, Illinois. Check 'em out.

VIII. Professional and Trade Associations

Professional associations often tape their seminars and make them available for very modest prices. They also offer a great deal of career-related literature. The Modern Language Association is a good example; it has a number of publications for liberal arts and humanities graduates, Ph.Ds, etc.

Strategy No. 2: Asking and Listening

Listening to people talk about their work has the advantage of two-way communication, an element missing from Strategy No. 1.

The good news is, the opportunity to employ this strategy is all around you—just for the asking. The next time you go into your bank, ask your favorite teller if you could discuss his or her job over lunch. (And don't forget to pick up the tab.) Chances are good you can find out about that job and the other jobs at the bank.

The key word is *asking*. Standing in line, you merely nod and say, "Two twenties, please" as your courage fails you. Not only have you missed an opportunity to learn, you have deprived the teller of the opportunity to feel good about his or her work. Or your travel agent. Or your family accountant. Most people are flattered to be asked for advice. People like to talk about what they do; it makes them feel good. And most people want to be helpful.

Some job seekers claim this method doesn't work, that people aren't willing to give the necessary time. From our experience, most people *are* willing to talk about their work if you demonstrate a sincere interest in what they have to say by:

- Coming prepared with well-thought-out questions.
- Actively listening to them as they talk.

A critical strategy here is to approach individuals with whom you have something in common. This is referred to as *networking* (networking will be discussed in greater detail in Chapter 4). Here are five resources you could tap for asking and listening about the world of work:

I. Relatives, Friends, and Acquaintances

Start with the obvious: your flesh and blood. Ask as many of your relatives as exist on the family tree to tell you what they do, where they work, how they actually perform certain tasks, why they selected their careers, what they like and dislike about their work, and what issues and problems they are facing right now, on the job. (Allow for plenty of time to catch up, if your relatives haven't seen you for a while.)

Close friends fall into this category, too. And don't forget about casual acquaintances, like ministers, priests, rabbis, school principals, mayors, bankers, and so forth. These individuals often have access to many people.

II. Fellow Alumni

A natural bond exists among fellow alumni, which explains the success of high school and college class reunions, alumni clubs, directories, college sports enthusiast groups, etc. Alumni directories—particularly those of professional schools, such as law, business, engineering, and the like—often contain not only addresses and phone numbers, but alumni places of employment and job titles.

III. Trade and Professional Associations

Almost every conceivable industry, trade, profession, or group of individuals sharing a common interest eventually organizes into an association. These groups hold regular business meetings, offer training and self-help workshops, hold annual conferences and trade shows, and publish trade journals and newsletters. Some even publish complete membership directories.

These associations are fair game for you, the labor market novice. Their very *raison d'etre* is for people to come together to exchange ideas, information, job opportunities, and industry trends. These get-togethers offer you a great chance to, yes, network: to ask the person sitting next to you what organization he works for, what position he holds, and how he got there; to buttonhole a speaker and ask her to give you the exact title of a book she mentioned during her presentation; to exchange business cards with vendors in the exhibit hall.

Many associations are organized at a local, regional, national, or even international level, and hold conferences at every level. Some even have subgroups organized around the issue of disability. Two examples are the disabled users group of The Boston Computer Society, and the American Psychological Association, which has an active disabled membership.

To locate the association of your choice, check out *The Encyclopedia of Associations* at—you guessed it—your local library.

IV. Other Blind People

No doubt one of your most prolific sources of employment-related information will be other blind people employed in your field of interest, or in a company where you would like to work. As a fellow blind person, they can speak directly to the issues which affect you in your job search (and later on in the job)—issues such as the attitude of the company toward minority persons, what alternative methods exist for doing the job, accommodations that the employer made, and problems with other employees, supervisors, and subordinates, and how they handled them.

Successfully employed blind individuals can serve as important role models. We, the blind and otherwise disabled, like women, blacks, Hispanics, and other minority groups, have discovered that as we progress up the socioeconomic ladder, it is helpful to have role models to consult and to inspire us as we make our way. The role models benefit, too. Being sought out for guidance and advice reinforces their self-esteem and confirms their elevated, and hard-earned, status.

Here are some ways to identify other blind individuals who are working in your field of interest:

(a) A potential gold mine of people resources can be found in any of the self-help organizations of the blind. Both the American Council of the Blind (ACB) and the National Federation of the Blind (NFB) serve as umbrellas to many special-interest groups, such as blind educators, lawyers, computer specialists, entrepreneurs, secretaries, and so forth. If you are a blinded veteran, you can contact the Blinded Veterans Association.

The JOB Project, a program jointly funded by the Department of Labor and the National Federation of the Blind, has the ability to generate people contacts across state lines.

(b) The American Foundation for the Blind (AFB) administers the National Technology Center, which has amassed a large database on blind people who are using computers on the job.

Another important resource is The Job Index, a national information network of blind people who are in competitive employment. AFB's Job Index contains over 600 names, including information on how people heard about, applied for, obtained, and are productively managing their jobs.

(c) The Project on Science, Technology, and Disability of the American Association for the Advancement of Science has compiled a directory of over 1,000 disabled scientists, engineers, and assorted other professionals. *The Resource Directory of Scientists and Engineers with Disabilities* is available in print for $10 plus $3 for shipping and handling.

(d) National Braille Press has published several computer books which list names and addresses of people using computers in various occupations.

(e) If you already own a particular piece of equipment, such as a paperless braille device or closed circuit TV monitor, you could contact the vendor and ask for names of other users, or join any of the users groups organized around specific equipment, such as the VersaBraille Users Group.

(f) The Greater Detroit Society for the Blind has published the *Occupational Information Library*, a compendium of descriptions of jobs performed by blind individuals.

(g) If you have a rehabilitation counselor, he or she should be able to provide you with names of contacts. Projects with Industry programs in your state may also be able to provide you with names of blind employees they have helped to place in competitive employment.

V. Talking to Employers
If you want to know more about a job, why not talk to employers themselves? Sounds logical.

This approach gained momentum in the seventies with the "informational interview." Career counselors theorized that while employers might be reluctant to talk to anyone whose clear purpose was to ask them for a job, they might be more willing to talk to someone who just wanted *information*.

This strategy evolved into the informational interview—a question-and-answer session with a knowledgeable employer, where you talk about major trends, job specifics, industry competition, job qualifications, and the best strategy for finding a job in the field.

By following such a strategy, job seekers were able to fashion a succinct job objective, target prospective employers, prepare a more focused resume, and impress hiring managers with their in-depth knowledge of the employers' needs.

Unfortunately, this strategy was poorly understood and widely abused. Thousands of job seekers descended on unsuspecting employers, asking for nothing more than an informational interview, "believe me." Once seated in the employers' offices and spurred on, no doubt, by the excitement of the moment, they would forget their purpose and blurt out, "Do you have a job for me here?" And so, the informational interview fell into disrepute, making it difficult for true practitioners of the strategy to use it.

Difficult, we said, but by no means impossible—*especially for blind job seekers*. As a blind job hunter, you have a distinct advantage in using this strategy to check out jobs.

Let's face it. Sighted people are curious about blind people. They just can't figure out how we do things. Use this natural human curiosity to your advantage. As a blind job seeker, you could call up an employer in your field of interest and say something like, "I'm blind and thinking of becoming a stockbroker, but I need to get a closer look at how the job is done so I can make adaptations. I need to spend some time with a stockbroker, such as yourself, in order to identify and discuss alternative ways of doing the job. Will you help me?"

How can they turn you down? You have just provided them with the unique opportunity to meet and talk with a blind person about how their job could be done by someone without sight. It's intriguing.

Just don't ask for a job. (And don't mention the words "informational interview.") Use this strategy the way it is supposed to be used: to get a closer, in-depth look at the job. And don't forget to take the time to discuss the alternative strategies you might employ to do the job. After all, that's your expertise, and that's the intriguing part you can offer the person who agreed to discuss the job with you.

Here's an example of how one of the seminar participants used this strategy to get a closer look at a particular occupation:

"I was one year out of law school, and a recruiter for a law firm made the mistake of telling me that his firm had once interviewed a blind law student but they couldn't figure out how he would fit in with the firm. I told them quite bluntly that if they really were serious about the possibility, they should fly me to Denver to talk to the firm about it. Their hiring season was over for the year, but my purpose was to go down and educate them, and educate myself about how I could work in a major law firm.

"To my surprise, they agreed. I spent two days discussing adaptations and approaches. I met some truly wonderful people, including a lawyer who had grown up on the wrong side of the tracks, so to speak. Chuck had known failure, and he valued perseverance. Two things happened. A friendship started which has lasted over a decade (and led me to some of the best watering holes in Denver), and after the two days were over, the law firm offered me a job.

"I didn't end up taking the job, because my law school dean assisted me in getting a clerkship in Los Angeles. Two years later, however, they did successfully recruit a blind associate into the firm."

It's not hard to identify people who may be willing to share specific job information with you in an informational interview. Here's how it works:

(a) Think of someone you know—a neighbor, clergy, relative, fellow Lion, or co-worker—who may know the person you want to meet, or who may know someone in your field of interest. This is the intricate process of making contacts, or *networking*.

Networking takes Stamina, Courage, and Gentle Persistence. Once mastered, it will be one of the most valuable skills you will ever acquire in your working life. There is a saying among career counselors that each one of us is never more than four or five contacts away from anyone we want to meet, including the President of the United States.

Why not contact the person directly, you ask? Because of another bedrock principle of human behavior: You will be more welcome if you are referred and recommended by a mutual acquaintance.

(b) Ask your contact to smooth the path for you by calling the person you want to meet, and to alert that person that you will be calling. Ask your contact to let you know when he or she has done so.

(c) Call your party, refer to the mutual contact, and set up an appointment for a date, time, and place of his or her choosing. Indicate that you only need 30-60 minutes, so he or she won't think you're going to take the whole day. People are busy. If you sense that the person would prefer to talk over the phone, graciously oblige, even though a face-to-face interview is preferable.

(d) Think through and write down specific questions; employers are easily frustrated by people who waste their time by coming to a meeting unprepared.

(e) Meet your party, take detailed notes, avoid small talk unless initiated by your host, ask for permission to telephone later if other questions arise, thank your host, and leave.

(f) Thank the person in writing. Do it the same day. That way, the person will be more receptive to future contact. Anyway, it's common courtesy.

Strategy No. 3: Observing

There are countless opportunities, every day, for observing people at work—the possibilities are as great as your imagination and courage.

If an insurance salesperson visits your home, you may buy her policy and then ask her to give you some information in return: How is the rate book laid out? How many calls does she make on an average day? What method of compensation does the company have? If she sold you a policy, you have already observed a salesperson at work.

The next time you book a flight with your travel agent, ask if you can come in and observe the work site. Notice how information about flights is obtained, and the manner in which information is relayed to customers. Observe the office environment: Is there a lot of joking around, or are things dead serious?

Contact the realtor who sold you, or your parents, a house, and ask to observe him at work. Notice what time he starts work and how much work is done after 5:00 p.m. Observe his manner with both customers and sellers; ask about salary and commission, and why he thinks he's a good realtor.

Write to your favorite radio announcer or disc jockey and ask for an appointment to come into the studio and observe. Ask about the equipment they use, and gather enough data to determine whether the equipment could be adapted for a blind person. Ask about their training and preparation for this type of work. Get a feel for the atmosphere: Is it really as fun-loving as it sounds on the air?

When you next visit your parent's place of work, watch one of the secretaries progress through a typical day's work—typing, filing, trying to read her boss's handwriting, taking dictation, taking messages, screening calls, sorting the mail, chatting with co-workers, making reservations and setting up appointments, welcoming visitors, making personal phone calls, and so on. You will learn much more about a secretary's job by observing her at work than you will by simply reading her official job description.

If you don't know anyone in a particular company you would like to visit, arrange for a guided tour. Call either the organization's public relations department, or better yet, contact a manager there. If the facility only accepts group tours, organize one.

Observation should not be a passive activity; you can make the most of it by actively analyzing the many facets of any job. Here are some tips for improving your powers of observation.

Six Ways To Improve Your Powers of Observation

1. Observe at least two people with the same job title, for several reasons. Titles mean different things within the same company, and from one company to another. For example, a secretary in one company may report to one person; in another, he or she may take assignments from three or four people. Some secretaries hold strictly clerical positions, while others may have considerable control over business matters.

Likewise, the title "manager" can mean something quite different, depending on the company, or even on the manager's individual style. Some managers bury themselves in the smallest details of every project, while others delegate the responsibilities and limit their involvement to a final "okay." (Incidentally, some say this describes the basic difference between Jimmy Carter's and Ronald Reagan's operating styles.)

Finally, some people puff up their titles a bit; it's human nature to want to inflate our status by using a more sophisticated job title and exaggerating our responsibilities.

2. Look at a job *in its entirety*. Some jobs are more repetitious in nature, like assembly line work, which might take 15 or 20 minutes to observe. On the other end are managerial jobs which are often highly complex and contain many component parts.

When you make arrangements to observe a job, ask how long it will take to observe the whole job. If you observe a manager's or a salesperson's job for only a few hours one day, you may be unlucky enough to catch the manager on precisely the afternoon he has chosen to seclude himself in the office to prepare the yearly budget, or the salesperson on the one morning of the month when she stays in the home office to compile sales records and plan calls for the next month. You may miss the manager in his role as coach, mediator, negotiator, or meeting chairperson, and you may miss the salesperson doing what earns her a living—namely, marketing, meeting personally with prospective customers, closing sales, and servicing accounts.

If you need help identifying the component tasks of any given job, consult the *Dictionary of Occupational Titles*.

3. Every job is part of a work flow. On an assembly line, it's easy to track the work flow, but more complex jobs demand closer investigation. Observe the job's relationship to and interdependence with other jobs, both inside and outside the organization.

4. We mentioned earlier the advantages of talking to blind employees, but don't fall into the trap of limiting your career options based on what other blind people are doing. This type of behavior—common among employers and counselors—has already frustrated many a pioneering soul. Let us, at least, free ourselves of this type of restrictive thinking and base our job options on our genuine interests and proven skills.

Another possible sandtrap, in terms of observing blind people on the job, is the unfortunate situation some blind people find themselves in where they are not given any real job responsibilities, but merely serve as the "token" disabled employee. In that type of situation, you will have to distinguish between what the person should be doing in that position versus what they actually are doing.

5. As you observe both blind and sighted people at work, begin to develop your own ideas on how you will handle these three important aspects of the job: (1) time management, (2) delegation, and (3) job adaptation.

Time Management. Study the time sensitivity of certain tasks. Some aspects of the job are more urgent than others. While you may need to read memos, letters, and messages as soon as they reach your desk, you may be able to postpone the reading of a report or resume until that evening or the following morning. This distinction is an important one for blind people who are looking at jobs that require a lot of reading and paper management. What may look like an overwhelming amount of paperwork could turn out to be quite manageable, with some planning.

Delegation. Learn to distinguish between job tasks that *must* be carried out by you, and those tasks that could be delegated to others. An attorney, for example, must read transcripts of hearings, prepare briefs, and argue cases in court. But he may assign the tasks of researching past judicial decisions and verifying the accuracy of citations to a paralegal.

Job Adaptation. Remember that choosing an alternative technique is a *personal* decision based on reading and writing preferences (braille versus speech or large print), financial resources, and technical aptitude. You may prefer to take braille notes during a meeting, or you may decide to memorize the main points of the meeting and commit them to paper once the session is over.

But more important, the adaptations you select should enhance your productivity. When you observe other people at work, analyze how you might be able to do those same tasks more efficiently. Ask yourself, "Can I really complete on an equal footing with my sighted co-workers? How? What equipment will I need? Will it mean working a little longer each day to get the job done? Am I willing to do that? What accommodations will the employer be willing to make?"

6. Every organization has its own culture and value system which are reflected in the company's management style, written policies, and unwritten traditions and practices. Study the organization's climate. Are senior executives addressed by their first or last names? Ask yourself, "How will my rather stiff, conservative nature fit into this loose, funky environment?" Or, "Could I tolerate this suffocating formality ten hours a day?"

Observe the company "perks" (benefits bestowed on higher-level employees, like offices with window views, first-class travel, executive dining rooms, company cars, etc.). Are these important to you? What influence do these perks have on the level of competitiveness among employees? In other words, look beyond the job tasks and study the whole work environment.

Tips for the Blind Young Adult

For sighted people, exploring the world of work can be a somewhat passive and incidental activity. From a very early age, sighted children unconsciously learn that work is one thing and leisure is another; they begin to notice the difference between formal work attire and after-hours jeans. Television and magazine ads bombard kids with images of work environments, with lots of clues about what goes on inside a plant or in a corporate headquarters.

As teenagers, they get a closer look when they work at a hamburger joint, run errands for their parents, or work temporarily at a gas station or as a secretary in their mom's company. They observe the janitor cleaning the hallways, the cop directing traffic, the firefighter at the scene of a fire, the store manager negotiating with distributors, and the cook at

McDonald's. They watch similar images on television, like *L.A. Law*, *Designing Women*, *Dallas*, and *Hill Street Blues*.

Then there are field trips to the farm, the coal mine, the airport tower, radio and TV stations, the stock exchange, or through Sara Lee's kitchens or the Hershey chocolate factory. In this way, sighted children are exposed to a fabulously rich and painless education about the world of work.

But for blind children and teenagers, education and exploration of this kind must take a more active "hands-on" approach, rather than the passive "looking on" experiences so easily available to their sighted peers.

Here are some ideas to help blind young adults familiarize themselves with the world of work:

1. Ask a parent or teacher to describe work-related images and scenes shown on television, in movies, at the theater, or in books, magazines, and newspapers. At the same time, inquire about work-related concepts, such as attire, working hours, the work environment, bosses, vacations, strikes, and so forth.

2. Ask a parent or relative to bring you to work with them periodically, to introduce you to colleagues, and to let you roam freely about the place. This, in itself, conveys a clear message that blind people, like sighted people, belong in the workplace.

3. Develop a curiosity for work-related objects: the look, shape, and feel of power tools, briefcases, typewriters, computers, uniforms, calculators, office furniture, paychecks, supplies, etc.

4. Actively participate in school-sponsored tours, or arrange your own (perhaps through a local chapter of a national organization of the blind). Try to expand the breadth of your experiences by visiting and getting the feel of as many different types of work sites and atmospheres as possible: agricultural, mining, manufacturing, sales and office locations; blue-collar and white-collar environments; urban, suburban, and rural

workplaces; smokestack as well as "clean" industries. Observe hard physical labor, technical skills, manual coordination, professional analysis, and executive decision making.

Talk with your teacher or parent before going on the tour about your need to touch and familiarize yourself with the layout of the plant, equipment, tools, etc. By the way, just because you have visited a plant once doesn't mean you shouldn't go back another time. Modern technology is affecting the workplace so dramatically that you might not recognize a plant from one tour to the next.

5. Ask a friend to walk down a busy street with you and describe every business on the block. Another way to do this is to go through the telephone business directory.

6. Visit the museums of science, technology, and industry in your city. And don't forget about the many expositions and trade shows that come to most big towns.

Strategy No. 4: Actually Working

Nothing takes the place of actually working.

By the time sighted students have completed their high school or college years, they have accumulated a number of on-the-job experiences, such as babysitting, mowing lawns, managing a newspaper route, pumping gas, packing grocery bags, or working as a camp counselor. In college, there may also be internships and co-op work experiences. The major motivator may be money, but the real reward is the *experience* of working.

Temporary and part-time work experiences give you a track record: You are a proven commodity, and no longer such a risk. And, as a blind person, you must be able to demonstrate to prospective employers that you can handle work responsibilities when you apply for full-time, permanent work. A chief executive officer at a mid-size bank put it this way: "I don't care how many degrees you have, if you don't have any work experience, we don't want you."

This feeling was echoed by a personnel manager at a high-tech firm: "The best advice I can give is to get some work experience. I don't care if it's volunteer or part of an internship. If you don't have any work experience, you're a risk, and employers shun risks."

Yes, it's the chicken-and-egg story all over. How can you get that precious work experience if no one will hire you because you lack work experience? Or because you're blind?

Traditionally, blind people have had a more difficult time gaining summer and temporary employment, for several reasons. Part of the problem is, of course, the employers' negative attitudes toward blindness.

The other problem is the fact that so many temporary jobs require working with equipment that would need to be adapted for a blind employee. Given the temporary nature of the job, and the possible expense involved—not to mention the time it would take to secure such a piece of equipment through the rehabilitation system—you can see that some jobs would be over before they could be adapted, even if the employer did agree to finance it.

Does this mean it can't be done? No. It means you have to be more selective and creative in your choices. It's more difficult. And while no one can guarantee that the situation for young blind job seekers will change overnight, the future does show promise.

Changes in the labor market will force some employers to become more flexible in their hiring practices. A good description of this change in the labor force appeared in a recent *Wall Street Journal* article entitled "A Shortage of Youths Brings Wide Changes to the Labor Market."

The article explained that because the birthrate fell sharply in the late 1960s and early 1970s, the number of people entering the job market today is smaller than a decade ago. At the same time, the number of new jobs is increasing, resulting in entry-level labor shortages, which translates into greater opportunities for those who traditionally have been left out of the labor market: the poor, the elderly, the handicapped, and immigrants.

Francesco Cantarella, a senior vice president at Abraham and Strauss, is quoted as saying, "Demographics will do more for equal-opportunity employment than all the government has done in the past six years."

Virtually all experts expect labor shortages to get worse before they get better. The U.S. Bureau of Labor Statistics projects that the number of workers between the ages of 16 and 24 will shrink 11% by 1990. Meanwhile, the number of jobs created between 1984 and 1990 will be a million higher than the number of people added to the work force.

A similar article appeared in *The Washington Post*, predicting that by the year 2000, 80% of all new entrants into the American work force will be *women, minorities, or immigrants*. Eighty percent! The article goes on to say that "demand is going to be enormous, and the demand for people with skills is going to be huge." Although the article doesn't specifically mention people with disabilities as a minority group, it stands to reason that employers will be forced to mobilize potentially qualified workers from every corner of the work force.

So, statistically, the labor market has never been better for young blind job hunters, seeking that important first-time work experience that will demonstrate to future employers that they can handle competitive employment.

Getting some work experience under your belt, as a blind job seeker, is even more important than it is for others. You have to prove to future employers that you can be a productive worker in spite of your blindness. Nothing is more convincing than demonstrating a proven track record, *before* graduation, which is when the job-search process begins.

A young blind man, who recently got a job as a programmer, got his foot in the door because he had had a paper route during high school. When the hiring manager heard that this blind guy had managed a paper route, he said, "Bring this fellow in, I want to find out how in the world he managed that!"

Here are ten strategies for finding part-time and temporary employment:

I. Personal Contacts

Every spring, millions of fathers, mothers, uncles, aunts, grandmothers, and grandfathers besiege their companies' personnel departments with inquiries about summer work for their sons, daughters, nephews, nieces, and grandchildren. Most requests are answered favorably; it makes sense for employers to hire the sons or nieces of trusted employees rather than gear up the expensive machinery for locating, interviewing, screening, and training total strangers for temporary work.

Here, again, the key is using your personal contacts. Spread the word that you are looking for summertime work among friends, relatives, colleagues, clergy, members of the local Lions Club, even members of the boards of directors of private agencies for the blind (they often run or own thriving businesses and, one would hope, have an interest in giving blind youngsters opportunities to demonstrate their skills and compete on an equal footing with sighted youngsters).

Here's how one seminar participant used his family and personal contacts to gain summer employment:

"I grew up on a farm, a chicken farm, and my summer employment was laid out for me. (Laughter) That was a very good experience because one aspect of the job was handling cash. We had a roadside stand and sold farm-fresh eggs. We did a lot of business because the main road led to Cape Cod. I was expected by my parents to sell the eggs and make change—my blindness was never an issue. I was a member of

38

a farm family, and there was work to be done. It was the most important experience of my life.

"Another job I had, during high school, which was very important for me, was trucking. A neighbor of ours had a trucking business, and I helped him load and unload. It gave me a feel for what the work was like, doing physical work like that all day.

"And another job I had during the summers of my college years was working as a part-time dispatcher for the police department. It was a very small town, and I had had some contact with the police. (Laughter) When the dispatchers took their summer vacations, I would fill in. Every one of these experiences was a very meaningful part of my future."

(Today this "farmer" is an international marketing manager.)

II. Your Elected Representatives

Approach your U.S. senators or representatives in Congress, your state senators and assemblypersons, county supervisors, city councilpersons, and members of the Community Planning Board. These elected officials and their aides not only have a natural desire to help their constituents, but are also very well connected. You will find many of them to be quite helpful with tips and information.

Also, some of them control a number of slots in certain prestigious internship programs, such as the Congressional Page program, the Congressional Intern program, and the State Legislative Intern program. Urban fellowship programs also exist, which are administered by municipal personnel departments.

III. Your Own Advertisements

We were surprised at the number of seminar participants who had placed their own ads to gain summer and part-time work. Here are some of their experiences:

"My parents had the philosophy, not just with me but with all of us kids, that you had to do it yourself—they wouldn't help us get jobs. So I put an ad in the newspaper to babysit, and I had tons of work all over the neighborhood."

(This woman is now a customer support representative for a computer company.)

"The same thing happened to me. I was in my sophomore year in high school and my friends were starting to get real jobs, like at Burger King and that sort of thing, and I had no money. If you have no money, it's a major hassle. The only jobs I could think of involved cash. So I complained to my father that there wasn't anything I could do, and my dad mentioned it to a friend of his. This man was in the newspaper business, and it was the Sixties and the space industry was booming. So this guy put an ad in the paper saying, essentially —I never saw it—'blind student looking for summer work.' He got several calls, and they made the selection at the newspaper!

"We didn't even know about it until one day I got a call, 'Can we come interview you?' Two guys came to the house to interview me; it was so embarrassing. But the only thing they and I could figure out was for me to type, so I got a job working for IBM that summer, typing 40 hours a week. I hated it, just hated it. But it was a good thing: It convinced me to go to college, because I didn't want to type for the rest of my life."

(Today this "typist" is the head of a consumer relations department for a large governmental agency.)

"I have a newspaper story, too. When I was getting ready for law school in the fall, I figured I really had to do something that would give me some idea of what was what, so I went down and talked to maybe 20-30 employers—without any success. We knew a lot of people in the community, my dad had a lot of contacts, so these weren't cold calls. But no one would give me a chance.

"In desperation, I sat down and got hold of the community relations editor for the local paper and basically blew my top in a letter, saying, 'Here you have a city agency serving the blind, and you probably have 80% unemployment among the blind in this community. You have people getting summer jobs through the mayor's city programs, and here I am, wandering around without any prospects.' I dared them to publish the letter. They did.

"I got a call from the mayor of the city the next morning, offering me a job. He said, 'I'd like you to come in. We have a job placement program where we place 5,000 kids for the summer. I want you to be my assistant, running that program.' And that's what I did. He said, 'What do you need to do your job?' And I said, 'What do you want me to do?' He replied, 'Well, we're hiring 5,000 kids this summer. You're going to need files on every one of them.' I looked up at him and said, 'Five thousand kids and I'm starting today. Great.' He gave me two reading assistants, whom he told me to go out and hire, and he said, 'Get going—that's the last time I want to see you for the summer.'

"The assistants and I stayed up all night brailling 5,000 cards; in fact, we spent the first five days doing that, but it worked out. Later, I did some legal work in the area and found the connections I had made there very useful."

(Today this fellow is an attorney with a private law firm.)

IV. Traditional Summer Jobs

Don't overlook the traditional paper route. We have heard of blind teenagers who managed paper routes because they possessed good mobility skills and took the necessary time to learn the routes (and where people wanted their papers put). It requires more time because you probably won't be moving on a bike, but it's doable.

The biggest problem you face is convincing a paper route manager to give you a chance. Here's a strategy that worked for one of the seminar participants:

"I went down to talk to the guy at the newspaper distribution office, but he said, 'Sorry, I'd like to give you a job, but I just don't think a blind kid can handle a paper route.' So I went home and talked my sister into signing up for the route. Then I took over the route, and several weeks later went back to that same manager and explained that I had been managing the route. It really did tickle him, the way I did that. Of course, I got the route. I hope that's the hardest job I ever have to do; it was really tough. But, then, I heard that from all the kids."

There are lots of neighborhood businesses that constantly require part-time help. Grocery stores, for example, always need packers. Packing is something you do with your hands, not with your eyes. Again, the trick will be convincing a reluctant employer to give you a chance. Offer to practice in the store after-hours. Better yet, start practicing at home by packing and repacking foods from your kitchen. Recruit a fellow student who has packing experience to explain the proper techniques to you.

Restaurants are always looking for people to make salads, cut up vegetables, or do odd jobs in the kitchen. Practice at home so that you can display an air of confidence when you step into a restaurant kitchen.

Companies that sell products need telemarketing people, like the photo studio down the street, or the local newspaper. Telemarketing offers you a chance to learn how to sell, an extremely important skill for almost any job.

If you possess good writing skills, offer to write a series of articles for the local newspaper on sports, hi-fi equipment, personal computers, food and restaurants, etc., for $15 an article. If you want to, you could use your expertise with a disability as your forte and offer to cover disability issues. Remember when women were only allowed to report on domestic topics, like cooking, entertaining, interior design, and fashion? Today they cover the gamut.

Many part-time job opportunities exist right in your own backyard. You can distribute "babysitter" fliers, organize a giant yard sale, make Christmas wreaths, or offer to do chores for elderly neighbors, like cleaning, shopping, shoveling, raking, or washing cars. You can place a notice advertising your services in the church bulletin, on a bulletin board at the Laundromat, or in the local paper. Offer the first three hours free to every new customer. People will view you as an enterprising young adult, which will help you when you contact them for job leads and references.

There is a fast-growing movement of young people—high school and college students—going into business for themselves. Such entrepreneurship demonstrates the ability to work hard, initiative, reliability, self-confidence—all the things employers love, if you ever plan to work for one. A good resource is the Association of Collegiate Entrepreneurs, based in Wichita, Kansas.

A resource book for summer jobs is *The Summer Employment Directory of the United States*, published by Writer's Digest Books of Cincinnati, Ohio. You can find it in most public libraries.

V. Volunteer Work

True, volunteer work won't pay the rent, but at this stage of your career, your primary concern is getting some work experience under your belt. Nonprofit agencies, like churches, synagogues, political groups, and hospitals, often can't afford to pay you because of serious financial constraints. Even so, you can turn a volunteer experience into a rewarding— perhaps even paying—position. That's what happened to this seminar participant:

"The most important thing for me when I got started was volunteer work. I turned a volunteer summer experience into a five-year employment opportunity after college. It was a group-home situation, with juvenile delinquents, and they needed volunteers who were willing to work for $50 a month plus room and board. Fifty dollars, if they had the money that month! I remember very carefully drafting a letter, between my junior and senior years in college, really selling myself and dealing quite openly with the issue that I was blind, and that I didn't have the slightest idea of how I was going to deal with a bunch of juvenile delinquents. (Laughter)

"But what I was doing was turning the tables. Here they were, out soliciting volunteers, and here I was, asking if I could please come work for them. So they were happy to have me, in spite of the fact that they didn't have any idea, nobody had any idea, what was going to happen. Later, of course, it turned into a full-time position."

Sign up to work on a political campaign. Campaigning involves a lot of community work, canvassing, telephoning, and so forth, which will increase your contacts. And if your candidate wins, don't forget to solicit his or her help in the future.

Another way to make volunteerism work for you is to use it as a strategy to gain entry into a company. You may encounter an employer who is able to pay you for your services but may not be convinced that you can do the job. Offer to volunteer for three months, on a trial basis. What does the employer have to lose? There should be some understanding that if you work out, they will consider you for paid employment.

Finally, use volunteer work to gain needed skills and test possible job adaptations. Volunteer experience always looks better on a resume than white space. Consider the volunteer programs administered by the Action Agency of the federal government, as well as the Peace Corps, and study the *Directory of Volunteer Opportunities* published by the Career Information Centre of the University of Waterloo, Ontario, Canada.

VI. Vocational Student Organizations

Students enrolled in vocational training programs are particularly close to the action; they study work firsthand. Check out some of the national organizations, like the Future Farmers of America, the Future Business Leaders of America, etc. They offer supervised occupational experience programs, where you might be assigned to a farm, for example, to study farming as a vocation.

VII. Internships and Fellowships

Internships are an excellent way to gain on-the-job experience. They exist in thousands of work settings, from art galleries to hospitals, from radio stations to consumer advocacy agencies. For a comprehensive listing, send for the *Directory of Internships* from the National Society for Internships and Experiential Education.

A number of major employers, aware of their legal obligation to employ people with disabilities, have established summer internship programs for students with disabilities. Perhaps the largest summer job program of this kind is administered by the David Taylor Research Center (a unit of the U.S. Department of Defense) of Bethesda, Maryland, which has employed hundreds of disabled students over the years in challenging assignments with excellent results.

Before you accept an internship, try to reach an understanding with your prospective supervisor about what you will be expected to do, and learn, on the job. Throughout the internship, schedule periodic sessions with your supervisor to review your progress, and to make sure you are, in fact, learning something of value.

Expect to do your share of "grunt work," such as filing, delivering messages, etc. Everyone does some "grunt work" along the way, and even low-level tasks offer valuable opportunities to learn about the organization's business.

Fellowships, like internships, also offer on-the-job learning experiences. One prestigious example of this is the White House Fellowship, established in 1964 to "provide gifted and highly motivated Americans with firsthand experience at the highest levels of government."

There are no educational nor professional criteria for application for a White House Fellowship. During a one-year assignment in Washington, DC, White House Fellows serve as special assistants to Cabinet secretaries or to senior members of the White House staff. In addition, the program offers extensive educational opportunities, including seminars with top government officials, eminent scholars, journalists, and corporate leaders. The program is administered by the President's Commission on White House Fellowships in Washington, DC.

For other sources of information about fellowships, contact the Foundation Center in New York City, or any of its collections of materials in major cities throughout the country.

By the way, if you are a student and looking for scholarship aid possibilities, try to identify fellowships and scholarships endowed by corporations. If you win a fellowship or scholarship of this kind, you will probably have an inside track with the endowing corporation, later, when the time comes for the company to select candidates for a limited number of summer job slots.

VIII. Co-op Work Experiences

Some colleges offer co-op work experience, where you can learn while you earn on the job. In other words, you alternate classroom study with paid work experience.

According to career consultant Joyce Lain Kennedy in her column "Co-op Education is Ideal Career Preparation," a co-op job, on the average, pays $6,500 to $7,000 a year and could lead to permanent employment after graduation.

She goes on, "Even if you don't stay with the company where you worked as a student, you'll have experience in the career field of your choice and thus will have an easier time landing your first full-time job.

"Co-op jobs can be highly responsible assignments. For instance, students work as daily newspaper reporters, use computerized spreadsheets to devise management tools for project planning, work in intelligence divisions of drug enforcement agencies, do preplacement health screenings and prepare toxicity reviews of chemicals used at production sites .... For free information, drop a postcard to the National Commission for Cooperative Education in Boston, Massachusetts."

IX. Temporary Employment Agencies

Temporary employment agencies offer an excellent means of "surveying the field," that is, moving from one assignment to another, from one company to another, checking out the possibilities. Temporary jobs exist for both blue-collar and white-collar workers.

Be forewarned, however, that most agencies won't know how to handle your "case," and will need a great deal of assistance from *you*. If you have a demonstrable skill, like typing, loading, packing, etc., you should explore this possibility in earnest.

Peggy Robinson, the Eastern Massachusetts area manager for Manpower, the world's largest temporary employment service (1,200 offices in the U.S.), says that in the 20 years she's been with the company, not a single blind person has come in looking for temporary work. She says they have had several deaf clients who have worked out well.

She also adds, "It would be great if qualified blind applicants came in for work. We need good people." When asked what kinds of jobs might be available for blind applicants, she said, "Bindery work, medical transcription, telemarketing, and receptionist positions are often available at Manpower."

To locate temporary employment agencies, check the Yellow Pages, or the *Membership Directory* of the National Association of Temporary Services in Alexandria, Virginia.

X. The Rehabilitation Agency

If time is running out, and you still don't have a summer job, contact your local rehabilitation agency for a job there. The reason we mention it as a "last resort" is that most employers will be more impressed if you have worked *outside* the blindness system, rather than for a rehabilitation agency where, they suppose, the work was somehow not as competitive. Nonetheless, you should consider every avenue open to you to gain work experience.

A number of rehabilitation agencies, Mayor's Offices for the Handicapped, and other similar organizations administer temporary work programs. These may have a variety of titles, such as summer employment, transitional employment, supervised work experience programs, etc. The transitional employment program of the Vera Institute of Justice's Project Job Site in New York City is one example.

Do's and Don'ts for the Temporary Worker

Once you have landed any temporary job, you have only a short time to impress your boss. Besides, you are being evaluated as a "disabled employee," which calls for extra finesse. Here are a few common-sense do's and don'ts for the first-time worker:

1. *Understand Your Assignment.* When your boss gives you an assignment, make sure you know what the boss expects in these three important areas: quality, quantity, and timeliness.

Learn to listen carefully and follow instructions. It's a good idea to repeat the assignment: "So you want me to . . . ." Managers sometimes get careless in their communications and forget to mention some very important details. Don't be afraid to ask for clarification—it's better to be right than sorry.

2. *Refrain from Giving Unsolicited Advice.* As a general rule, don't offer to "straighten out this mess around here" as a temporary worker. Although things may not look organized (and maybe they're not), there may be good reasons for the way things are being done. If you want to make a suggestion, present it as a hypothetical "Do you think it would work if I . . . .?"

3. *Make Job Adaptations Easy.* It's a rare employer who would invest much time, energy, and money in a temporary worker in terms of job accommodation. It just doesn't pay.

It's better to say, "Hire me, and I'll pay for my own readers" (even if it amounts to your entire paycheck) than it is to expect the employer to make the investment for a part-time or temporary job. Such an approach shows that you are serious about the job. Employers respect that; employers like motivated and gutsy people who really want to work. Show them you do.

4. *Get Acquainted with the Personnel Department.* During lunch, stop by the personnel office and make yourself known. Find out about their job-posting system, and let them know what you're looking for—remember that insiders generally get the first shot at in-house job openings.

5. *Show Enthusiasm for the Job.* Attitude and approach are two big words in the world of work. Nothing, other than raw talent, will affect your boss and co-workers more than your overall disposition. Be vivacious rather than indifferent, enthusiastic rather than disinterested.

Do more than is expected of you; don't just sit idly until you receive the next assignment. Always be on the lookout for opportunities to help.

6. *Get an Evaluation of Your Work.*   Toward the end of your summer internship or work assignment, ask your boss for an "exit interview." An exit interview is an opportunity to candidly discuss your performance, what mistakes you may have made, how you could have done a better job, and what additional skills or training your boss would recommend.

Many supervisors will have difficulty giving honest feedback if it's negative. They may feel badly about your blindness and may not be able, emotionally, to discuss your weaknesses. Or they may think your weaknesses are a result of your blindness.

It is to your benefit to insist that they discuss both your assets and liabilities. Explain to your boss that such feedback is the only chance you have to improve your work and be better prepared for your next job. Lead them into the discussion by asking probing questions: "How did I handle this . . . or that?"

Be sure to get your boss's home and work addresses and phone numbers for future contact. You may need a letter of recommendation for a permanent position later on.

Tips for Parents: Preparing Your Blind Child for the World of Work

Your attitude and the expectations you hold for your son or daughter will greatly influence their eventual participation in the work world. You can begin to instill a healthy self-image in the mind of your blind child at an early age by:

1. Demonstrating to your child that there's "more than one way to skin a cat." More often than not, there are many ways to accomplish a task and achieve the same result. For example, while a sighted child may cross the street safely by *watching* oncoming traffic, your blind child may cross the street equally safely by *listening* to traffic sounds. While you can *see* the flame coming out of the stove, your child may *feel* its heat by holding his or her hand over the burner. And while you may use a pen and paper to take down a name or phone number, your child

may use a braille slate, a braillewriter, a pocket cassette recorder, or simply memorize the information.

Openly discuss with your child the advantages and disadvantages of various options, and encourage your child to develop an analytical, problem-solving approach to the world around him or her. Such an approach will help your child devise alternative techniques in the workplace, later on.

2. Teaching your blind child to avoid making false assumptions and inappropriate comparisons to sighted people. If, for example, both your child and a sighted friend knock over their glasses of milk, explain that the milk was spilled because they were both clumsy, not because one of them is clumsy and the other is blind.

Explain that the fact that a sighted person may *theoretically* be able to perform a certain task that a blind person couldn't (and vice versa) is meaningless. What *is* significant is whether the sighted person actually *can* perform the task or has any interest in doing so. Having sight may be a crucial requirement for working as a surgical nurse, airline captain, or bus driver, but if the slightest drop of blood turns the sighted person's stomach, if he or she is terrified of heights, or has no patience for stop-and-go traffic, sight becomes irrelevant and the comparison loses meaning.

The ability to think clearly about such comparisons will help your child later in life as he or she argues for, say, a promotion before a possibly prejudiced line manager.

3. Helping your child to distinguish between a task that is well done and one that is not so well done. The issue of quality is an important one in this society. Convey to your child that it's not enough to simply complete an assigned task; one must complete it *on time*, *accurately*, *neatly*, etc.

Obviously, you will want to encourage your child in a positive, supportive manner about anything he or she accomplishes, but while sighted children, as they grow older, can begin to see the differences between the quality of their school projects and that of the other students', your child will need to learn about these differences through discussion.

4. Talking to your child about the fact that all human beings come into this world with both strengths and weaknesses. Talk about how blindness can, at times, be a problem, but at other times can actually be a plus, or of no consequence at all, depending on the situation. The bottom line for everyone who wants to be successful is to maximize strengths and minimize weaknesses. It is precisely this combination of strengths and weaknesses that makes blind people "normal" and "equal." None of us is free of handicaps.

5. Always encouraging your blind child to broaden his or her repertoire of capabilities and to learn new skills. It's a fast-changing world out there. All children need to be prepared to deal with new situations and unstructured environments if they plan to compete in the labor market.

6. Encouraging your child to be curious about the world (most children naturally are) and to adopt a can-do, problem-solving approach to life's dilemmas and everyday difficulties. Classes in science and technology should motivate your child to ask how things work. Sit down and figure out ways of doing things which, at first, look impossible because your child is blind. If you can teach your child to adopt a positive approach to these challenges, he or she will have a much better chance, later in life, of succeeding in the workplace.

Recently, some creative ways have been devised for children and adolescents to learn about the business world in general, and, more specifically, about how some individual businesses function.

One example of this is The Stock Market Game, sold by the Securities Industry Association, which teaches high school students about trading shares and investing in the stock market. Whatever occupational field your child is interested in, inquire of the professional society or trade association related to it whether they sponsor educational programs for young people.

A more ambitious program can be found in the banking field. The Young Americans Bank, located in Denver, Colorado, was founded in 1987 as the nation's first bank to cater to children and teenage customers. In addition to processing the transactions of its young clientele (the average age of its savings account holders is nine), the bank conducts an extensive program of educational seminars and workshops for youngsters under age 22 about such topics as investing, obtaining credit, and managing bank accounts.

7. Finally, making sure you enroll your blind child in schools which have a strong orientation toward career education and exploration. A growing number of public schools are beginning to establish close working relationships with local corporations. Some classes are even being taught by senior managers, and individual children are paired off with mentors from the participating companies. What a wonderful way to begin learning how to network.

The California Foundation on Employment and Disability, of Manhattan Beach, California, is a consortium of Los Angeles area high schools and corporations which conducts a program of this kind, called High School/High Tech, specifically for severely disabled students. At least one other consortium, in the suburban Washington, DC, area, is in the planning stage.

WHAT TO EXPECT
FROM THE WORLD OF WORK

As you reflect on your work experiences, you will gradually begin to understand what a strange, exciting, and complicated place the workplace is. You will observe many personalities, attitudes, and vested interests. You will notice patterns of behavior that are at times consistent, and other times not. You will observe human motivation at work, sometimes rational and sometimes not.

You will learn that sighted people, just like blind people, vary greatly. Some may be quite willing to give you a fair shake; others will never get used to your blindness. Some supervisors will expect you to be as productive as your sighted co-workers; others will shelter you from the work load.

Over time, you will discover that there are as many management styles as there are personalities. Some supervisors are authoritarian, and jealous of their prerogatives; they may be less willing to listen to advice from subordinates. Others may openly encourage your participation in decision making and readily share information about the management process. Some managers promote a spirit of rivalry and competition among their subordinates; others encourage a more cooperative atmosphere of teamwork.

You will begin to notice an unspoken distinction between the formal reporting channels and the informal relationships between people, between the way things are *officially* supposed to be done and the way they *actually are* done.

You will learn that no relationship is more important than the one you have with your boss. The more work experience you gain, the more adept you become at "managing your boss," and the more job satisfaction you will enjoy.

Finally, you will begin to understand what "office politics" means. You will see some people politicking for small stakes, covering their own mistakes and sabotaging other people's work for petty self-aggrandizement. You will see other people politicking for high stakes, pursuing exposure and visibility in hopes of promotion and greater power. In the process, you will learn when to hold your tongue, and when to go to the mat.

You will discover that while technical knowledge can and does play an important role in the hiring process, it's often the personal chemistry between the applicant and the hiring manager that actually determines who gets the job or the promotion.

Understanding the world of work comes with experience—the experience of reading, asking and listening, observing, and actually working.

It's a lifelong education. ¤

Chapter 2
Assessing Who You Are
and What You Can Be

Their bitterness filled the room. Eighteen successfully employed blind people sat around a large conference room table, talking about their frustrating experiences looking for challenging work. Their anger reflected the lack of guidance, support, and encouragement they had received from those around them.

One seminar participant recalled her frustrating experiences looking for her first job:

"It was the summer between my junior and senior years in high school. I went to the local rehabilitation agency and said, 'I'm planning to go to college in another year and would like to have some summer work experience.' The first thing they threw at me was, 'How about a vending stand: wet or dry?' I said, 'Neither, thank you, what about a job that will teach me something about office work?' They just wouldn't yield. They suggested proofreading and darkrooms. I refused both. I told them what my skills were: teaching and working with children. I suggested some type of summer school program with kids. I said, 'What about my bilingual skills? I'm fluent in Spanish.' No way.

"Finally, I went to my mother, who worked at Children's Hospital, and asked her for help. I ended up working for the summer in the emergency room, doing translating work for anyone who came in off the streets and spoke only Spanish. It was a tremendous learning experience. I learned to keep file cards, how to handle complete strangers in an emergency situation, and how to deal with hospital personnel, not to mention the fact that I developed a network of contacts that I used later on."

Other seminar participants had similar experiences, dealing with other people's limited expectations of them:

"No one knew what to do with a blind person, in terms of work, so I was encouraged to stay in school. And if you're blind and going to college, you're expected to major in things like rehab, social work, or special education . . . and then you just get in deeper and deeper. You get out and work for a state agency, and by the time you've realized that you have other interests, no one wants to hire you because you've been with the state agency for too long."

* * * *

"I'm working on my third career right now. First was unemployment, the second was working as a vocational counselor, and now I'm into computers . . . .

"The problem for me, in terms of self-assessment, dates back to high school. At that time, I was a good student and my interests were in the hard sciences—physics, chemistry, and mathematics. And who did I have around me to help assess my potential in this area? Peers, parents, guidance counselors, and people like that. I was discouraged from pursuing a field I really love. I was told by significant others, 'Let's be realistic: What about social sciences? It's still science, you know.' And at that point in my life, what did I know about the working world? It didn't matter how well I did in school, I was seen as a blind kid, and blind kids couldn't do physics, even though I was getting all As in it at the time .

"So here I am, almost 12 years later, finally getting back to the hard sciences. Why? Well, now it's okay for a blind person to go into computers. But the real reason is that I finally believe in myself. I'm making decisions for myself now."

* * * *

One way to evaluate our skills is to rely on the feedback we receive from others. In this area, too, people with disabilities often receive inappropriate feedback on their behavior and abilities, as these seminar participants explain:

"Of course, your own family's attitude can color your own self-assessment. Either they over-applaud your accomplishments, or they expect very little, which also affects your sense of self. Sometimes it takes years to uncover who and what you *really* are, compared to anyone else. We all know blind people who think they're hotshots because everybody has been telling them they're wonderful just because they get out of bed by themselves. I recently had that kind of experience. A friend of mine and I did a reading of Proust—he did it in French, and I did it in English, reading from braille. He got a few compliments, but I was so embarrassed when everybody came up to me and told me how great I was."

* * * *

"Even grades aren't necessarily an objective assessment. So you get an A on an essay test; maybe it's because your instructor feels sorry for you.

"What I've been doing lately is trying to find objective measures of my own performance compared to others in the field. I've been asking people who sell radio air time about quotas; what do they normally run in a given month? I don't tell them I'm asking for myself, because the automatic response would be that I couldn't do it. I ask around, like I'm just curious. If I get a sales figure that seems way off, I check out the person's standard of living. If it seems to be higher than others', I recognize that this person is at the top of the scale. Or, if he drives a beat-up car, maybe he's lying about his sales figures. I'm trying to get an idea of what the standards are so I can compare my potential performance objectively, for myself."

* * * *

"That's good. I like that. Another way to think about standards and ways of objectively measuring our performance is to look at those of us here today. All of us were invited because we have successfully managed our way into the labor market, working productively and happily, I hope. What do we share in common? One, this is a highly verbal group. Two, most of us are extremely assertive. And three, I would say we are 'deviant,' in that we won't take 'no' for an answer."

* * * *

Some of the more interesting comments regarding self-assessment, had to do with blindness-related skills:

"I think we share more than that. I want to bring up the issue of mobility with respect to self-assessment. Everybody in this room got here by themselves. Nobody held their hands, they didn't come with their mothers, they didn't come with their brothers, they came with their dogs or canes—their eyes. The first thing that has to happen, before you can get a job, is that you have to have the confidence from within to get around independently—just as automatically as a sighted person walks down the street, drives a car, or takes public transportation.

"If you don't reach that point in your self-confidence, never mind about getting a job. If you can't walk down the street to the drugstore, none of these other things we have been talking about will take place. Uncle Harry may line up a job for you, but if you have to walk in with your mother, you're finished. That doesn't mean you can't ask the security guard for some assistance, like where's the elevator, but it means, overall, that you've got to get around on your own. Mobility is the first step toward higher self-esteem."

* * * *

"I agree. You could be the next Einstein, but if you can't get around, you don't make a good impression—either in your eyes, or in others'. I learned mobility when I was ten years old. I was encouraged, very early, in a public school situation, to be as independent as possible. Frankly, I think that's what guided me along the path to everything else. I could do the same things my classmates did. I could go get a pizza, I could take public transportation downtown, go shopping, I could do all these things. Later, I never questioned whether I could get to an interview or the local library to do some job research. You have to have confidence in yourself, to be able to walk into a room, find a table, and sit down."

* * * *

"As you said, and I agree, for any of us to compete in the job market, we must have a certain degree of mobility. But we must also be literate, which means using braille and other technologies to read and write. Those skills earn parity for anyone competing in the labor market. And that means we must also learn to use the *most efficient* means of reading and writing, even for taking notes. It's not enough to be able to do it; you must be able to do it efficiently. The goal is to be as versatile as possible in one's skills."

These comments point out the additional difficulties faced by you, the blind job seeker, in sorting through the hodgepodge of emotions and expectations of others to find a career direction that really matches your personality, values, and skills.

Unconsciously, you may adopt the prejudices of others and come to believe that "chemistry might be possible for a partially blind person, but never for a totally blind person," or that because all of your teachers are sighted, teaching must require sight. Or, because most of your rehabilitation counselors are blind, that that must be a good field for blind people.

The current types of jobs that are being touted as "good for blind people" include taxpayer service representative for the IRS and computer programmer. For some people, these jobs are a good match. For others, they hurt like a bad-fitting shoe. Both are sedentary, and require an attention to detail which may excite one person and drive the next to delirium.

The argument has been: But isn't a job—any job—better than no job at all? That's for you to decide, but remember that your decision will affect the rest of your working life, which is a long, long time. Before you jump on the first job bandwagon, ask yourself carefully, "Is this the right job for me?"

Being pigeonholed into certain occupations is an old story for women and minority groups. True, many minorities accepted "suitable jobs" as an entrée into the work force, but if you talk to those people today, you find that many people wish they had struck out into new territories—even at the risk of rejection and discriminatory treatment. It's always worth a try.

At least recognize that you may be pursuing a career path influenced by subtle (or not so subtle) discrimination. A popular anecdote from the Sixties shows how this can happen. Ben was a young black kid who, on his way to school each day, passed the neighborhood cop (who was white), the local storekeeper (who was white), the construction foreman (who was white), and the street cleaner (who was black), arriving at school where his teacher was white and female. One day the teacher asked Ben what he wanted to be when he grew up. He replied, "A street cleaner." The teacher cringed. "Why?" Ben replied, "Because I know I can do it."

Discovering what you can and want to do, unencumbered by such prejudices, is a hard task. How can you define your own set of skills, needs, and interests, rather than falling back on what is socially "appropriate," allegedly "feasible," or reportedly "available" to do? This chapter should help you learn how, but first let's look at why the process of self-assessment in general is so difficult.

WHY SELF-ASSESSMENT
IS SO HARD

Analyzing oneself in terms of a career, or even in general, is no easy task because:

¤ Human beings are naturally complex. If we were such simple creatures, psychotherapists, psychologists, and social workers would be out of business.

¤ Most of us are not accustomed to looking at ourselves introspectively, trying to uncover our basic values, innermost needs, and subconscious motivations.

¤ It's tough to be objective about such a subjective topic: who we are. And if we're blind, the truth may be even harder to get at, because others may not be honest with us.

¤ Most of us tend to define work-related skills and interests very narrowly. Since we have always compartmentalized our lives into *working hours* that are income-producing, on the one hand, and *non-working* or leisure time, on the other, we have come to believe that some of our skills and interests are strictly work-related and others are not.

¤ We, as blind people, have often been denied equal opportunities in education, training, and employment and have simply not experienced the world of work to the same extent as our sighted peers, have not tested ourselves in a variety of employment situations, and have not had the chance to study and evaluate our own reactions to diverse work environments. Consequently, we have not reached any firm and reliable conclusions about ourselves as workers.

Having said all that, self-evaluation remains the single most important task you face in your lifelong career exploration. Until you go through the painful process of uncovering *who you are and what you want*, you're not ready for your first career assignment.

Every career book on the market gives the same advice to job seekers: **Know thyself**. The problem is, most people think they can take shortcuts—just find a job and see how it goes.

You can, but chances are good, unless you're very lucky, that the result will be less than the best. We assume, if you're reading this book, that you want to do the necessary work to get the right position for you.

While this book does not attempt to replace the many good, practical guides on the market today that help you assess your skills, interests, and values, here are three possible strategies for self-assessment and vocational choice. All three strategies are based on different learning styles. Educators discovered long ago that some people learn best in a highly structured setting, that others prefer to design their own curriculum, and that some people work best with a combination of the two.

The first strategy for self-assessment is the **Reflection Pool**. The Reflection Pool is a mirror image of your life, past to present. It reflects those aspects of your life that hold significance and offer clues to potential career interests. This exercise will be introspective and stimulating for some; for others, it could be as laborious as a term paper. Read through the exercise and decide if this approach will work for you.

The second strategy is a self-paced workbook, **Creating Careers with Confidence**, written by Edward A. Colozzi and available for $10 from National Braille Press. This workbook is more structured than the Reflection Pool, but still highly creative. We will describe it in more detail, later in this chapter.

The third strategy uses a highly structured technique: **computer-assisted self-analysis**! There are several software programs on the market today that help you go through the process of defining your skills, interests, and values in relation to specific careers. The computer asks you certain questions, you provide the responses, and the computer analyzes the results.

You can begin the first strategy right now by continuing with this chapter. Here's how it works.

Self-Assessment Option No. 1: The Reflection Pool

How do you identify your skills, needs, interests, and values?

One way is *to record and analyze your past.* It's sort of like writing your own autobiography for the purpose of discovering what topics and types of people draw your attention and excite your curiosity.

Looking into your personal Reflection Pool gives you a factual basis for drawing some valid conclusions about yourself, because, whether you realize it or not, you *do* know, deep down inside, what excites you and is important to you. The hard part is bringing it to the surface. With a detailed history in front of you, the task becomes manageable—even fun.

Before your palms begin to sweat at the very thought of sitting down for hours at a braillewriter or typewriter to write a book about yourself, remember that this is *not* a term paper about to be graded by a fastidious instructor. This is not the time to worry about syntax, vocabulary, punctuation, or paragraphs. You are trying to do one thing: To unlock your past, to record it, and to analyze it in terms of your interests, skills, and values.

If you prefer, don't write it down at all; talk into a tape recorder. And don't feel compelled to complete your autobiography in one sitting. In fact, you should spread it over several working days or even weeks. Between sessions, as you go about your daily business, keep your memory roaming freely over your entire life and, as recollections surface, go to your braillewriter, cassette recorder, or typewriter and make notes.

Step One
Recording Your Reflections

Unlock the secrets of your past by reflecting on activities, achievements, or disappointments that meant the most to you and, consequently, could point you in a career direction.

Start talking or writing about each of the areas listed below. Record what you did and how you did it, what factors made you successful, what obstacles stood in your way, and what strategies you employed to overcome them. As you write or dictate, describe your emotional reactions to each situation, to the circumstances in which you found yourself, to the people around you, and to your own behavior.

For example, if fishing is a meaningful activity in your life, don't brush it aside as "play." Think about some possible reasons why fishing is so enjoyable, *e.g.*, because it's a solitary activity, because it gives you quiet time to reflect, because it's a sport, because it involves a particular skill, and so on.

Review these areas of your life:
- Paid as well as volunteer employment;
- Education from kindergarten through the highest level completed and adult education;
- Vocational and skills training;
- Cultural pursuits;
- Hobbies and crafts;
- Sports and recreational activities;
- Vacation-time experiences;
- Periods of rehabilitation and training in the skills of blindness;
- Civic involvement in political campaigns, social and self-help organizations, special-interest groups;
- Awards and commendations;
- Religious activities;
- Family and social relationships;
- Periods of poor health, incapacity, and hospitalization;
- Overall successes and failures.

Remember, though, in order for this strategy to work, you must be honest. No one else will be reading or listening to it, so be critical, but don't be afraid to blow your own horn, either.

Step Two
Identifying Patterns and Trends

Once you have recorded the key events in your life, begin to identify patterns, trends, and recurrent themes.

Which topics constantly draw your attention? What talents do you repeatedly demonstrate? What weaknesses in your education, training, and personality tend to appear and reappear in your autobiography? What experiences do you obviously enjoy? What type of organization or association do you, as a rule, prefer to work in, join, or patronize? What kinds of people are you drawn to?

Be careful not to generalize. You may conclude that working for a governmental agency is not for you because you had a negative experience working for one. Closer reflection points to the fact that an overbearing supervisor was the real culprit, and not necessarily the environment.

After you have recorded and identified trends in your personal Reflection Pool, there are five more steps to the process.

Keep going, you're doing fine.

Step Three
Uncovering and Prioritizing Your Interests

As you identify the events in your life that reveal to you what your interests are, strip away the distinction between work and play. Everything you do, day or night, reflects your interests. While it's true that only a handful of baseball, skiing, sculpture, and movie buffs turn their interests into paid employment, it's also true that entire industries surround recreational activities and employ thousands of people in hundreds of occupations.

Today, people are increasingly looking at careers they would *enjoy*. The recent trend toward career switching, job-hopping, and entrepreneurship stems from our need to find more satisfying work, based on our interests and not just our abilities. You hear about the cosmetics marketing executive who goes windsurfing every weekend and suddenly abandons his corporate career to open a windsurfing equipment and supply store at a sunny beach resort. Or the engineer who quits his high-paying position to open an inn in Vermont. Or the rehabilitation counselor who spends her off hours dabbling in computers and finally shifts to a career in a computer software firm.

The benefit of closely examining your interests is the possibility of landing a satisfying position the first or second time around, rather than waiting half or—mercy—all your working life.

Some people never get there.

If your goal is long-term career satisfaction—and it should be—you need to identify and *prioritize* those interests that are reflected in your life history so far. If you adore soap operas, chocolate, or your trip to England, let these interests help you identify potential job opportunities. You could write a soap opera, teach English literature, or open a gourmet chocolate importing business.

You might. But would you want to?

In order to move from general interest areas to possible career options, you need to question whether your love of these things is *so great* that it could sustain you in a lifetime career.

How can you find out?

Part of the answer lies in the difference between "liking" something and "being bewitched" by it. Bewitched is the computer buff who cannot wait until the clock strikes five to run home and "work" all night on a database. She reads every kind of magazine and newspaper article on the subject, and what she doesn't know, she finds out. If a new computer terminal is announced, she writes away for the literature; if a new printer is being demonstrated, she is there to test it, see it, touch it, and listen to it. She shops by computer, banks by computer, communicates with friends—even total strangers—by computer, and plays games on a computer. This is what really "turns her on." And this is what *you* want to tap into in your career exploration.

Take time now to define and prioritize your interests, as reflected in your life pool.

Step Four
Defining Your Skills

The next step in the process is to define your skills. Skills? Oh, my, I don't have any skills. Yes, you do. Even babies have skills; they can grasp objects, push and pull, sit up, and, most important of all, smile.

You have some skills you probably don't even think about, like reading braille, traveling with a white cane, memorizing numbers, or using a tape recorder or braille printer. These skills may, in fact, be some of the most important job-seeking and on-the-job skills you possess. How about your volunteer activities in organizations of the blind, which involve a number of useful skills that can be transferred into a work environment?

If, for example, you are an active member of the American Council of the Blind, the Blinded Veterans Association, the National Federation of the Blind, or any other consumer organization of the blind, you may have learned and perfected many skills that could be transferred into the labor market.

Recruiting new members is not so different from selling insurance, real estate, or mutual funds. The product is different, but targeting prospects, collecting information, persuasion, and follow-up are all essential elements of the selling process.

Likewise, you may have done some public relations work: writing and sending press releases, holding press conferences, preparing advertisements, and designing display booths. Add to this the abilities you have acquired in the process of organizing and conducting seminars, editing the organization's newsletter, raising funds, chairing meetings, lobbying the city and state legislators, and supervising volunteers, and you already have a good head start on your skills inventory.

To help you assess your skills, you can divide them into three categories: **specific**, **transferable**, and **personal**. Here's how you distinguish between these three skill groups.

1. **Specific Skills.** Specific skills are those skills that belong to a particular job, profession, or organization in which they are practiced. The technical knowledge and practice of law, for example, belongs to lawyers and the legal profession. Medicine belongs to doctors and the medical profession. The same goes for accounting, plumbing, computer programming, drafting, cooking, and so on. Each job requires *a body of knowledge* which, for the most part, is specific to that profession and cannot be transferred into other jobs. It generally requires courses of study or apprenticeship.

So, too, every organization has its own way of doing things, which may not be transferable to another setting. A newly-hired employee at Bank A has to learn "how we do things around here," including how the mail is distributed, what the dress code is, how the bosses are addressed, when performance evaluations and raises take place, etc. These are specific skills related to that organization or company.

2. **Transferable Skills.** No matter what kinds of activities you have been involved in, you have acquired some transferable skills. Do you possess writing and public speaking skills, negotiating and sales skills, the ability to prepare and interpret statistical data, management and supervisory skills, or manual dexterity skills?

Defining transferable skills, for some people, is difficult. If you are not sure what constitutes a "transferable skill," read through the following list taken from the *Dictionary of Occupational Titles* (DOT), which is published by the Government Printing Office and is available at your public library.

DOT Transferable Skills Listing

Career counselors have found it helpful to divide job skills into categories, depending on their relationship to **data, people,** and **things.** Some use a fourth category: **ideas.** Accounting clerks and computer programmers, for example, would be listed in the "data" category; rehabilitation counselors or kindergarten teachers would be listed in the "people" category; and carpenters or mechanics would fall under "things."

Here's how the *Dictionary of Occupational Titles* breaks down these skill categories, starting with DATA. (The skills are listed in order of *decreasing* skill level, from the very complex down to the simplest task in that basic category. For example, in the first listing, "synthesizing" is a more complex skill than "comparing.")

DATA		PEOPLE		THINGS	
0	Synthesizing	0	Mentoring	0	Setting-Up
1	Coordinating	1	Negotiating	1	Precision Working
2	Analyzing	2	Instructing	2	Operating-Controling
3	Compiling	3	Supervising	3	Driving-Operating
4	Computing	4	Diverting	4	Manipulating
5	Copying	5	Persuading	5	Tending
6	Comparing	6	Speaking-Signaling	6	Feeding-Offbearing
		7	Serving		
		8	Taking Instructions-Helping		

Use these skills categories to produce your own transferable skills list. For specific definitions of these skill areas, consult the *Dictionary of Occupational Titles*.

Be honest with yourself. Career evaluation is dependent on an honest appraisal of our skills.

3. Personal Skills. If you picked up this book, turned to this page, and only read the next sentence, it would almost be worth the price of the whole book. *Nothing is more important to your career and job-search success than your personal skills.*

Examples of personal skills include poise, self-control, honesty, charm, sensitivity, warmth, integrity, sense of humor, empathy, enthusiasm, responsiveness, cooperativeness, energy, self-confidence, and so forth. They encompass such personal qualities as manners, attitude, style, and approach.

Personal skills are employed by the doctor at your bedside, by the substitute teacher whose class is out of control, and by the salesperson who is empathetic to our needs. The presence (or lack) of appropriate personal skills may be more important to a successful job outcome than specific or transferable skills.

As we mentioned earlier, you may have a distorted view of your skills, based on less-than-honest feedback from the sighted world around you. To realistically assess your skills requires more than the usual effort; you will have to sort through your experiences very carefully.

Once you have analyzed your specific, transferable, and personal skills, you are halfway there. The critical other half of the process involves an assessment of the *strength* of these skills.

Step Five
Assessing the Strength of Your Skills

Just how good are your skills, really? Can you deliver what you promise? How do your skills compare to others'?

Few of us can claim to be the best at anything. Few of us are the worst—well, unless you consider singing. The nagging question remains: Just where do we stand on the spectrum between the worst and the best? How can we know? How do we evaluate ourselves if our parents and friends distort the picture, either by claiming that we have better skills than we do, or by underestimating our abilities? Furthermore, how do we assess our skills when our work experience is so limited?

Let's look at how an improper assessment of our skills can affect our career goals. Take the case of Mike Penn (a fictitious person). Mike wanted to leave his job as a taxpayer service representative, and upon reflection, decided to pursue a career in writing. He had written a play in the fifth grade that his mom thought was terrific. Recently an article he wrote on computer access for the blind appeared in a publication and received good reviews. He decided he would become a technical writer. After all, he had purchased a computer the year before and had taught himself several programs, and he possessed good English skills.

Mike designed a resume, highlighting his writing experience—limited as it was—and attached the article he had written for the computer magazine, in its original state, pre-edited, because he didn't agree with the changes the magazine editor had made. He got the names and addresses of several computer companies and sent out his resume and cover letter. And then he waited. And waited. And waited. Nothing happened. Ever.

Mike concluded that technical writing wasn't for him. In the fall, he entered law school. Maybe Mike will be a fine lawyer, but he'll never know if he could have been a thriving technical writer, and enjoyed it more.

Why did Mike fail?

For one thing, he failed to evaluate his writing skills *compared to others in the field*. He paid no attention to the competition, and how their qualifications compared to his. Two, his ego destroyed any other chance he may have had with the clipping he sent—pre-edited. Three, he had no idea what additional educational training might be required for technical writing. And, four, he did not persevere; he got discouraged after just one non-response.

Here are some things Mike could have done. He could have kept his job as a taxpayer service representative while attending night classes in technical writing. That would have given him a chance to try it out, in a non-threatening environment, and to solicit feedback from his professor about his chances in the field. He could have requested an informational interview with some technical writers, and asked for an evaluation of his writing, along with some tips about job prospecting.

The fact is, Mike did not properly assess his skills in relation to the competition, nor did he work to improve them. Nor did he have a realistic assessment of the working world. You don't have to make the same mistakes. You must aggressively identify and critically evaluate your skills—even more than most sighted people do—because you will encounter questions about your abilities because of your blindness. You can't assume that your skills are good, or bad, without a more rigorous evaluation.

If you believe no blind person can read braille faster than 250 words per minute, your whole perception of braille skills changes the minute you observe a blind court reporter reading braille at a speed of over 400 words per minute, as happened at a recent convention of the National Federation of the Blind. Everything is relative, including your skills.

Here are some strategies for evaluating your skills:

1. *Listen to What Others Say.* Leaving your relatives out of this for a moment, think about what other people praise or criticize you for. Try to distinguish between what a great job you did "as a blind person" and what a great job you did, period. Look for specific comments which may be more telling, such as "You

seem to have a knack for fixing broken machines," "You always remember names; I wish I could do that," "You sure have a way with numbers, pets, people, machines," etc.

2. *Seek Advice About Your Skills.* Ask others to evaluate a particular skill of yours. Reassure your evaluator that you are prepared for criticism (you'll have to be very persuasive), as well as praise. Insist that they be honest. Explain that only honesty will help you in the long run. Even in the short run.

Ask for specific and detailed criticism; don't accept vague generalities. For example, if you ask a friend, supervisor, or professor to critique a presentation you have just given to a group, don't be satisfied with a pat on the back and "It was great!" Rather, look for more helpful information, like: "What, specifically, was terrific about my speech? Could you hear my voice throughout? Did I look at the audience enough?" Only detailed responses of this kind will really help you evaluate your performance, perfect your skills, and determine if they are marketable.

But remember, John Q. Public, generally speaking, won't be able to offer criticism easily. Most people are uncomfortable confronting a blind person because of their feelings of pity. It's a fact of life. The best way around this, other than your powers of persuasion, is to select people whom you have known for a while, and who can offer honest feedback without these biased sentiments.

3. *Look for Credible Signs of Your Proficiency.* Getting a book accepted for publication is a credible validation of your writing skills. Getting a few articles published in mainstream magazines proves you're on the way. And being asked to speak at a large international conference tells you your speaking skills are good enough for you to get paid for them.

If you're handy with your hands, consider whether the machine works after you fix it. That's an objective evaluation—provided it didn't take you months to do the job.

Before moving to the next step, take the time now to assess the strength of your specific, transferable, and personal skills. Don't scrimp on time. This is important.

Step Six
Understanding Your Value System

This is the last part of your self-assessment exercise, using your personal Reflection Pool. It's a big one. It's about your value system.

Values loom large in our lives. Your "value system" is that combination of factors that you hold dear, the things in life that mean the most to you, like family, or money. The person who exercises religiously, quits smoking, eats no salt or sugar, not even chocolate, probably values good health.

We don't think much about our value systems, but values run deep. Any time you find yourself in a situation that conflicts with your values, you'll know—intuitively—that something is wrong.

It's time to take a good, hard look at your values. What do you value in a good relationship: loyalty, honesty, companionship, love, consistency? Is status important to you, or is helping your fellow man or woman your purpose in life? Does foul language bother you? Do you crave intellectual stimulation? These values, and many more, directly affect job satisfaction.

If you value family life, you may be happiest working in a family-like environment. If status makes you feel good, you should pursue a career in a highly visible corporate setting. If you care a lot about good health, you might quit your job as a systems analyst at a cigarette company for a comparable position at a health food chain. If improving society is a high priority for you, you would probably be more satisfied working as a publicist for the American Cancer Society than for a firm on Madison Avenue. Is a fat paycheck worth the insecurity of working for an aggressive, upstart computer software company? Are you going to be happier with the job security you get working at the post office?

Some of your values may be related to your disability. For instance, you may not tolerate working for a company where you, as the only blind person, are subject to demeaning attitudes from some co-workers, and feel a constant need to prove yourself. You may be more comfortable working in a blindness agency where, you would hope, attitudes are more progressive, or at least where people are not so uncomfortable in your presence.

You may value your independent mobility, which causes you to seek employment on a public transportation line, rather than depend on rides from co-workers. You may feel more comfortable working for a major corporation or government agency that provides paid reader assistance and technical devices, rather than working in a small company with a lean budget, where you have to scramble for your own resources. Maybe your values tell you that you want to work in an organization that has a generous medical benefits plan to relieve you of the financial burden of caring for your deteriorating eyesight.

You can't fool your value system. When things don't "feel" right, your values are probably being compromised. Rather than find yourself in such an unhappy situation, you should think about your values beforehand, and consider them a very important part of your career evaluation.

Of course, the more experience you have in living and working, the easier it becomes to identify values. If you have worked in both government agencies and private corporations, you have experienced the different "value systems" within these work settings, and how they affect you.

Some people, after working for a number of government and not-for-profit agencies, want desperately to move into the private sector, believing that the climate in most nonprofits is stifling, restrictive, and boring. Other people move from the private sector into the public sector because they want less emphasis placed on the bottom line, more job security, and more room for creativity.

Your values may even affect your working relationship with your boss. You might prefer constant direction from a supervisor, or you may rebel against anyone who "tries to tell you what to do." You may prefer to plan and implement your own projects, or you might prefer to be part of a team. Values identification comes only through constant and intense self-observation, and introspection.

As you begin to sort through your own value system, using your personal Reflection Pool, consider some of these factors:

¤ Values transcend your work life. Look at all aspects of your life, including your leisure-time activities, for values clarification.
¤ Values may be in conflict with one another. Your desire to travel may be in conflict with your love of family. Moreover, your values may be in conflict with theirs. While the job of your dreams is 50 miles away, your spouse's workplace is 50 miles in the opposite direction, or your elderly mother is in a nursing home 100 miles away, or the best education for your children is in another school district.
¤ No work situation will perfectly match all of your values; you must *prioritize* them. Start with the "absolute musts" at the top, and end with "nice, but not necessary." Recognize that any career decision you make requires some compromise, some trading off of values and benefits.
¤ The older you become, the more likely your values will have changed; some may disappear altogether. This is the healthy and normal process of maturation. When you were a roaming bachelor, you chose to live in an urban area blessed with an abundance of public transportation. Later, as a happily married man, you chose to move to the suburbs, where you sacrificed independent mobility for the social opportunities offered in a carpool arrangement.

A final word about values. Many people and events influence our value systems. If our parents think nothing is as important as money, we may internalize this value, or reject it outright because it came from our parents. A traumatic event in our lives, like a serious illness, may lead us into a career in health care.

In light of these various influences on our value systems, we must be prepared for constant change. We and the world around us are constantly changing. To survive, we must continually question and probe ourselves to determine how this affects our lives. We must plan for change. Part of that planning process is knowing yourself, and what you want. One participant at the employment seminar put it this way:

"Twenty years ago, my self-assessment would have been a lot different . . . things have changed around me, and my self-assessment fluctuates and changes with the times. There's a lot of information out there that I don't know today, but I might know tomorrow, and that would change my mind. What I tell you today I don't like, I might like tomorrow. You can't make up your mind who you are and end it there. It's an ongoing, ever-changing process. The best thing is to experience as much and learn as much as you can in as many places as you can."

Step Seven
Matching Your Interests, Skills, and Values With
Specific Jobs and Occupational Groups

Now that you have identified and evaluated your interests, skills, and values, you are ready to ask perhaps the most critical question in the entire career planning and job search process: In what job(s) or occupation(s) can you make use of your unique combination of interests, skills, and values?

Some of you may be fortunate enough to have already found your answer through your exploration of the world of work, which you did earlier.

First, you read about the world of work; next, you questioned both sighted and blind peple who are employed and discussed their work with them; after that, you observed people at work, and, finally, you actually landed and completed one or more temporary work assignments. In the course of all that activity, you may have hit upon your vocational choice. If you did, you may wish to proceed immediately to our discussion of the resume.

What if you still haven't settled on a career field? Is there a strategy which will assist you with a more comprehensive review of the world of work and lead you to some intelligent and logical decision? Yes, there is. And you'll be surprised at where you'll find it: Enter the federal government.

The U.S. Department of Labor publishes three books that are designed to help you through your predicament. These are:

1. *The Guide for Occupational Exploration*. It was last published in 1979 and costs $14.00.
2. *The Dictionary of Occupational Titles*. It was last published in 1977 and costs $23.00. Its 1986 supplement costs $5.50.
3. *The Occupational Outlook Handbook*. It is published biennially and the 1988/89 edition costs $22.00 in softback and $24.00 in hardback.

All these volumes are available from the Superintendent of Documents, U.S. Government Printing Office, Washington, DC 20402-9325. You should, of course, also check with your local public library. Although these are not the type of books which your librarian will normally allow you to take off the premises, you can ask, just in case.

The Washington DC Volunteer Readers for the Blind (WVRB) has recorded the 1986-87 edition of *The*

Occupational Outlook Handbook, and is planning to record the 1988-89 edition of the handbook, too. These recordings may be available at your regional library for the blind and physically handicapped.

These books don't read like novels. They are reference books, to be selectively researched and studied. Each of the three volumes has its unique purpose. Since you should familiarize yourself first with the *Guide for Occupational Exploration*, we'll describe it in detail for the purpose of motivating you to check it out.

The Guide for Occupational Exploration

The Guide for Occupational Exploration is a user-friendly reference work which is written in simple, nontechnical language. This is a feat in itself. In a single volume, this guide succeeds in providing the labor market novice, who has not yet settled on a career choice, with a precise and succinct description of all the *types* of work that exist in the American economy, and it does so in terms of people's personal interest in specific subjects.

We have decided to give you a sampling of what you would find inside *The Guide for Occupational Exploration*. Stick with it; we promise you, it will be worth your time.

The Guide for Occupational Exploration divides the entire world of work into twelve major interest areas. Each of these interest areas is, in turn, divided into a varying number of work groups. All together, the twelve major interest areas are divided into sixty-six work groups, which are further broken down into a varying number of subgroups. Each subgroup contains the titles of jobs.

To begin with, here are brief, one-sentence characterizations of the 12 major interest areas:

TWELVE MAJOR INTEREST AREAS

1. *Artistic*: Interest in creative expression of feelings or ideas.
2. *Scientific*: Interest in discovering, collecting and analyzing information about the natural world and in applying scientific findings to problems in medicine, life sciences, and natural sciences.
3. *Plants and Animals*: Interest in activities involving plants and animals, usually in an outdoor setting.
4. *Protective*: Interest in the use of authority to protect people and property.
5. *Mechanical*: Interest in applying mechanical principles to practical situations, using machines, hand tools, or techniques.
6. *Industrial*: Interest in repetitive, concrete, organized activities in a factory setting.
7. *Business detail*: Interest in organized, clearly defined activities requiring accuracy and attention to detail, primarily in an office setting.
8. *Selling*: Interest in bringing others to a point of view through personal persuasion, using sales and promotion techniques.
9. *Accommodating*: Interest in catering to the wishes of others, usually on a one-to-one basis.
10. *Humanitarian*: Interest in helping others with their mental, spiritual, social, physical, or vocational needs.
11. *Leading—Influencing*: Interest in leading and influencing others through activities involving high-level verbal or numerical abilities.
12. *Physical Performing*: Interest in physical activities performed before an audience.

Merely by reading through these 12 one-sentence characterizations, you probably already feel drawn to one or more of these interest groups. Fine, but your analysis has only just begun!

Each of these one-sentence characterizations is followed by a one-paragraph description of the kind of work involved in that interest area, the types of skill required, the typical setting in which the work takes place, and so forth.

Here is one example of a one-paragraph description under 7. Business Detail:

7. BUSINESS DETAIL

An interest in organized, clearly defined activities requiring accuracy and attention to details, primarily in an office setting. You can satisfy this interest in a variety of jobs in which you can attend to the details of a business operation. You may enjoy using your math skills. Perhaps a job in billing, computing, or financial recordkeeping would satisfy you. You may prefer to deal with people. You may want a job in which you meet the public, talk on the telephone, or supervise other workers. You may like to operate computer terminals, typewriters, or bookkeeping machines. Perhaps a job in recordkeeping, filing, or recording would satisfy you. You may wish to use your training and experience to manage offices and supervise other workers.

As we mentioned earlier, each of the twelve major interest areas is divided into a certain number of work groups. Here, for example, are the titles of the work groups under 7. Business Detail:

BUSINESS DETAIL: Administrative detail; mathematical detail; financial detail; oral communications; records processing; clerical machine operation; clerical handling.

The beauty of these work groups is that they help you focus on exactly what you want to do in the world of work. For example, if you have a leaning toward clerical work in an office environment, you may decide your skills are oriented more toward clerical machine operation, rather than oral communications.

Fortunately, each of the work groups listed in *The Guide for Occupational Exploration* has an excellent, two-page, detailed description of typical job activities, training requirements, work settings, and, best of all, clues which help you realize how your past interests and experiences may be related to the skill requirements of that work group, and indicative of your likely success.

Here is one example of a work group description under Business Detail called Oral Communications:

BUSINESS DETAIL: ORAL COMMUNICATIONS. Workers in this group give and receive information verbally. Workers may deal with people in person, by telephone, telegraph, or radio. Recording of information in an organized way is frequently required. Private businesses, institutions, such as schools and hospitals, and government agencies hire these workers in their offices, reception areas, registration desks, and other areas of information exchange.

1. *What kind of work would you do?*

Your work activities would depend upon your specific job. For example, you might:
- interview people and compile information for a survey or census.
- give information to bus or train travelers.
- operate a telephone switchboard.
- register hotel guests and assign rooms.
- prepare reports and insurance-claim forms for customers.
- receive callers at an office and direct them to the proper area.
- use a radio to receive trouble calls and dispatch repairers.
- register park visitors and explain rules and hazards.

2. *What skills and abilities do you need for this kind of work?*

To do this kind of work, you must be able to:
- speak clearly and listen carefully.
- use personal judgment and specialized knowledge to give information to people orally.
- communicate well with many different kinds of people.

- change easily and frequently from one activity to another, such as from typing, to interviewing, to searching in a directory, to using a telephone or a radio transmitter.
- use eyes, hands, and fingers accurately while operating a switchboard or computer keyboard.

3. *How do you know if you would like or could learn to do this kind of work?*

The following questions may give you clues about yourself as you consider this group of jobs.
- Have you participated in a school or community survey? Do you enjoy meeting and interviewing people?
- Have you given directions to others for finding your home? [have they able to follow your directions?]
- Have you had speech courses? Do you have a clear speaking voice? Do you use good grammar?
- Have you operated a CB radio? Do you like to use the equipment?
- Have you been involved in a communications unit of the armed forces? Would you like to continue doing this type of work?

4. *How can you prepare for and enter this kind of work?*

Occupations in this group usually require education and/or training extending from thirty days to over four years, depending upon the specific kind of work. People with a good speaking vocabulary and who like contact with the public usually enter these jobs. Some jobs require typing or general clerical skills. On-the-job training ranging from one month to two years is usually provided. Many employers prefer workers with a high school education or its equal. Chances for promotion are improved with additional education and training. Jobs in the federal government usually require a civil service examination.

5. *What else should you consider about these jobs?*

Often the worker may have to ask for information that is considered personal or confidential. People may have an unfavorable attitude about giving this information.

Workers may be assigned a wide range of duties, depending on the size of their company.

If you think you would like to do this kind of work, look at the job titles listed on the following pages. Select those that interest you, and read their definitions in the *Dictionary of Occupational Titles.*

§

Rather than continue to reprint the information which you can readily find in the *Guide*, we suggest you check out this valuable resource for yourself.

The *Guide* does not provide descriptions of the jobs themselves. This mission is accomplished by the *Dictionary of Occupational Titles* and its supplement. To help you make the transition from the *Guide for Occupational Exploration* to the *Dictionary of Occupational Titles*, the jobs listed in the *Guide* are each accompanied by a nine-digit code, which is identical to the nine-digit code which accompanies the corresponding entry in the *Dictionary*. For detailed research and study, you must work with the *Guide for Occupational Exploration* and the *Dictionary of Occupational Titles* in tandem.

But don't forget about the *Occupational Outlook Handbook.* This handbook contains full-length descriptions of some 200 high-density jobs (that is, jobs with large numbers of workers in them, most of which require at least some formal training and preparation).

The 200 jobs listed in the handbook include not only a description of duties and responsibilities, but also an outline of working conditions, an assessment of available opportunities, data on earnings, and occupational forecasts which predict whether a particular occupation is expanding, stable, or in decline.

Be careful about using occcupational forecasts, though, as a means of determining what fields of interest to pursue, or avoid. The fact that teaching jobs will be plentiful over the next decade is not a good reason to pursue a career in secondary education—unless you have carefully determined that that is the right career move for you. Occupational forecasts are as tenuous as weather forecasts. One minute it looks like sunshine, and the next minute it's raining on your parade.

That's because labor market changes are often triggered by unforeseeable events. The oil embargo by the Organization of Petroleum Exporting Countries (OPEC) in 1973-1974 created an overnight demand for petroleum engineers, geologists, and other experts in alternative sources of energy. Ten years later, the dramatic plunge in world oil prices resulted in a sudden glut of oil industry-related scientists, engineers, etc. No one could have predicted these changes.

Local market changes are unpredictable, too. The shutdown of Three Mile Island, the move of a major corporate headquarters, or the building of a large manufacturing plant in a farm community all shift employment patterns. The best way to discover what you want to do is to study work and assess your needs and skills. These three guides can help.

As you use these reference works, keep a couple of points in mind. First, use the introductory sections to make the most efficient use of these reference works—otherwise, it's slow going. Second, remember that with the world of work in a constant state of flux, some of the material will be dated. Third, use these reference works in conjunction with the other strategies mentioned previously, like talking, observing, and actually working. If you read about a particular job in the *Guide for Occupational Exploration* which you never heard about before, network among your friends and relatives until you locate someone who is employed in that field.

Finally, none of these reference works was written with the blind in mind; you will have to make your own adjustments to the text, and consider alternative techniques for handling the job tasks.

Self-Assessment Option No. 2: The Career Workbook

If you find you just can't sit down and look into your personal Reflection Pool, then you might want to try the self-paced workbook approach to self-assessment.

We have a specific workbook in mind, which takes much of the information available in the reference works mentioned above, plus an understanding of how skills, interests, and values affect job satisfaction, and puts them all together in a painless exercise book which you can complete at your leisure. The workbook is called *Creating Careers with Confidence* by Edward A. Colozzi.

Ed Colozzi is a dynamic, creative, and experienced career/life counselor based on the island of Oahu, Hawaii. He showed up at the National Braille Press one day, workbook in hand, wanting to know if, per chance, we had any interest in converting his workbook into braille for blind job seekers. Subsequently, we came to believe in angels.

Not only has Ed used his workbook with blind job seekers in Hawaii—with good results—but he even agreed to improve it and make it available as a supplement to this book. The result is a valuable, even enjoyable method of exploring your career options, based on your skills, interests, and values.

After completing a series of exercises in the workbook, you end up with a code that you can match up with with a job cluster at the back of the book. Here's what a typical job cluster looks like:

Applied Arts (Written and Spoken). Advertising copywriters; disc jockeys; legal assistants; advertising account executives; interpreters; reporters; public relations workers; lawyers; librarians; technical writers.

The workbook takes 10-20 hours to complete, but it's self-paced, which means you can pick it up and put it down at your pleasure. National Braille Press has produced a braille edition for $10. Print copies of the original workbook can be ordered from Delta Rainbow.

Self-Assessment Option No. 3: Computer-Assisted Self-Analysis

An astonishing amount of information about the world of work is now available on computer. But, of course.

These career exploration programs are called computer guidance systems. They provide users with an array of occupational and labor market information, including ways to prepare for occupations, the requisite skills, licensing requirements, information on post-secondary educational programs, two- and four-year colleges and licensed proprietary institutions. Some programs even provide career ladders and other useful tips.

Here's how they work. You sit down at a computer loaded with one of these career guidance systems, and interactively answer questions about your skills, interest, and values. (Yes, even the computer appreciates the importance of values.) Once you have answered all the questions (you can skip around if you want), the computer takes all this important information, analyzes it, and prints out those fields you might work best in.

One basic problem with these systems for visually impaired users is their excessive use of graphics—no doubt intended to keep sighted users alert. We know of one state agency, the

Oregon Commission for the Blind, which is making one of these computerized guidance systems accessible through speech. Since access for visually impaired users is not readily available across the country, you will need to entice an interested sighted friend or relative to go through it with you, reading the questions aloud. If you are familiar with a standard computer keyboard, you can tap in your own responses.

But don't let this discourage you from trying out one of these guidance systems. There are six major systems on the market today, and you generally can find them in high schools, career counseling centers, and universities. Here are three of the more popular ones.

The Career Information System (CIS) was developed in response to the need for a single, efficient information source that would relate career opportunities and decisions to post-secondary educational choices. Although CIS was developed in Oregon, all of the information is localized for any given state by a CIS staff located within that state.

Clients complete an introductory questionnaire that allows them to match their interests, aptitudes, and personal preferences with prospective occupations. For example, a "Descriptive File" contains information on several hundred occupations representing over 90% of the jobs in that state. A "Preparation File" contains information about preparing for that particular career, *i.e.*, skills requirements and licensing requirements, and a cross reference to appropriate post-secondary educational training. The "Program and School Files" provide information on post-secondary educational programs in that field, including two-year and four-year colleges and licensed proprietary institutions. You can even obtain a hard-copy printout of some of this information.

Another popular guidance system is **The System of Interactive Guidance and Information**, also known as **SIGI** (and now, **SIGI+**). It was developed by the same folks, at the Educational Testing Service in Princeton, New Jersey, who prepare those beloved SATs.

SIGI+ can help you figure out what you want from a job, and what you have to offer to the world of work. It can get you facts about occupations and put the pieces together to help you make a career decision. One thing SIGI+ tells you it *can't* do: "SIGI+ can't go out and hunt for your next job." Well, computers do have their limitations.

If you already have an occupation in mind, you can ask SIGI+ for more information about skills, training, job outlook, etc. It can give you a job description of a typical job, in detail, including salary. Once you complete the self-assessment exercises, you can call up certain occupations and ask why they would, or would not, be the right match for you. The answers can be surprising.

DISCOVER is another sophisticated career guidance system. It comes in several versions, ranging from grade level/high school versions to college/adult learner versions, and even specialized versions for business organizations and the military. The system is marketed nationally through the American College Testing Program (ACT) offices, and is designed on the premise that career development is a process that takes place throughout a lifetime.

DISCOVER lets you browse the ACT World-of-Work Map, which simplifies career exploration by grouping more than 12,000 occupations into 23 job families and 12 map regions according to their involvement with data, ideas, people, and things. This map is similar to a large pie, divided into 12 pieces, and you can receive hard-copy printouts of any of this information.

Before we leave the subject of career assessment, we should caution you about using any type of "quick fix" to solve a problem which demands prolonged introspection—as the process of self-assessment does. That's why so many people, after completing a one- or two-hour vocational interest test, are shocked to learn they should go into acting or the ministry. Who, me?

The process of evaluating what you can and would like to do in the world of work takes time. These self-assessment "tests" are helpful tools, but they should not be used as a substitute for hardcore self-study and analysis.

WHEN ALL ELSE FAILS

If none of these three self-assessment strategies work for you, then you should enlist the services of a professional career counselor. Career counseling services are offered at little to no cost by college and university career planning and placement offices, and by a variety of community organizations, religious institutions, and individuals.

Once again, check references and make certain that your prospective counselor's beliefs and assumptions about blindness are positive.

TOUGH ANSWERS FOR TOUGH QUESTIONS

Once you have identified, prioritized, and evaluated your interests, skills, and values—phew!—you are ready to move on to the next stage of your job search. If you don't complete this process of self-evaluation, it will haunt you for the rest of your working life.

We promise.

The process of self-assessment never ends. You need to continually examine your internal set of expectations. How will you measure your success on the job? What expectations will you set for yourself? Are they realistic? How driven are you to perform the job on the same level as your sighted co-workers? Can you? Will you be competitive? How can you measure your output, your productivity, compared to others'? How does your disability affect your job performance?

These are tough questions. They require tough answers. You need to begin to develop a philosophy about how you, as a blind employee, will compete in a sighted world. You need to because, you can be sure, the employer will be thinking about it—and looking for the right answers, from you. ¤

Chapter 3
Your Personal Calling Card

Imagine sitting next to Frank Perdue on a first-class flight to Hawaii. In the midst of a lively conversation about his phenomenally successful promotion of chickens—plump, juicy chickens—he puts the challenge to you. He promises you unlimited money to finance your job-search campaign, with the sole stipulation that you successfully draw attention to your product: you.

Thinking over your alternatives, you imagine your svelte, physique striking a fanciful pose on a king-size billboard overlooking Hollywood Boulevard . . . or your tough investigative style filling in for Dan Rather . . . your name gracing a sports column in *The Washington Post* . . . better yet, your picture on the cover of *Fortune* magazine with the caption, "Meet One of America's Savvy Business Minds."

This nonsensical conjecture reveals the secret of packaging your product: Identify your strong points and then find the best way to get them noticed. Regardless of what you've read, no one prescription works for everyone. You are one of a kind, and there are countless ways to promote yourself in the job market. Look at what Frank Perdue did for the common chicken.

WHAT IS A RESUME?

A resume is a self-advertisement. It is a tidy, enticing advertisement of yourself, and it must pass the flash test—those first *30 or 40 seconds* that the reader gives it before tossing it into the nearest trash can. If you doubt this, consider the fact that large companies receive over 200,000 resumes a year; even small companies get a dozen or so a week. To pass the flash test, yours must stand out from the rest.

"The underlying assumption," says Tom Jackson in his book *The Perfect Resume*, "is that if you can't communicate about yourself in a way that invites interest and attention, you aren't fully equipped to deal with today's highly communications-oriented work world."

How you present yourself on paper is indicative, in the minds of employers, of how you present yourself to the world. Are you careful or sloppy, clear or disorganized, verbose or succinct? And, most important of all, are you oriented toward results? After all, results are what employers care about. What you *did* is not as important as what you *accomplished*.

This chapter is intended to supplement—not replace—the many books and guides on resume preparation. Your local library will be able to recommend a few of the more popular ones; study them. This book will examine the resume as the personal calling card of a *blind* job seeker, and the implications that deserve your attention. Here are a few tips:

1. *Be Creative and Flexible*

Stop thinking of resumes in cookbook terms: such-and-such a length, your work history in reverse chronological order, no personal information, typed on a certain kind of paper stock, and so forth. In the history of job hunting, jobs have been offered to people with "perfect resumes" and to people with no resumes at all, to job seekers with one-page resumes and to people with six-page ones, to job hunters who openly flaunt their blindness, and to those who make no reference to it at all. Tailor your resume to the specific job you are applying for—and learn to be flexible. In these times of word processing and PCs, this is easy to do.

2. *Stand Out from the Pack*

Think for a minute about the person on the other side of the desk: the recruiter. Faced with an endless pile of resumes on his or her desk and a quickly approaching deadline, do they painstakingly read through each and every resume? Do you believe in miracles?

Resume reading is a screening process. Recruiters take this mountain of paper and quickly, very quickly, *skim* through the pile, looking for a sentence, a phrase, some word that coincides with their idea of the best candidate. The goal is to find a *few* qualified candidates to screen in—the rest are screened out.

In this environment, you must do whatever you can to stand out from the pack, to impress your prospective employer with the fact that although on paper you may be no better (perhaps even less striking) than your competitors, you are different enough, uncommon enough, interesting enough to merit a closer look. You are a person worth meeting face-to-face.

3. *Be Selective*

Resumes were never meant to be comprehensive life histories. Pick and choose only those aspects of your past history that convey a positive image of you. It's a matter of *emphasizing* and *de-emphasizing*.

Does that mean you can lie? Absolutely not. But you can pick and choose those elements of your life history that will convince a prospective employer that you are a likely candidate for the job and worth meeting.

A resume is like a product advertisement. Before advertisers bring a product to market, they painstakingly decide which product strengths to promote, and which failings to play down. You should use the same strategy to sell *your* product.

But they aren't supposed to lie. You shouldn't, either.

4. *Demonstrate Your "Product"*

Musicians, on-air broadcasters, designers, and other entertainers and artists have always known that a demonstration tape or portfolio of their work offers the best—and most convincing—proof of their talents. This strategy is not limited to artists and entertainers.

Press releases and brochures serve the same purpose for public relations professionals, schematics for architects, a speech translated from English to Japanese for translators, a legal brief for lawyers, and so on. This approach also works well for career changers who don't have a chronological work history to support their new field of interest.

If you are a teacher, for example, and you want to join a training and development department in a major corporation, you can send a training packet along with your cover letter. If you're a carpenter, welder, electrician, or work with your hands in some other way, bring in a product that represents your workmanship and dexterity, or have a photo taken of it and mail it with your cover letter.

The point is, sometimes a traditional resume either does not offer the best proof of your skills (as in the case of musicians) or works against you (as in the case of a teacher wishing to change careers). In those circumstances, some tangible proof of your skills may be preferable to a resume.

Clearly, this approach will help you stand out from the sea of traditional resumes surrounding most personnel professionals. It draws attention to your product . . . remember Frank Perdue.

5. *Target Your Resume*

Sending your resume out willy-nilly to the attention of the personnel department can be an exercise in futility. To understand why, let's look at why personnel departments exist, and what they can do for you.

People in personnel act as advisors, assistants, and facilitators on personnel matters to the people who actually carry out the business of the organization: the line managers. People in personnel, generally speaking, have no authority to make final *hiring* decisions on behalf of line managers.

They can, however, and do influence the hiring process by drafting job descriptions, setting pay ranges, identifying potential candidates inside and outside the organization, preparing recruitment ads, communicating with employment agencies, college placement offices, and executive search firms, screening incoming resumes, pre-screening candidates through interviews, and submitting *short* lists of potential candidates to line supervisors for them to interview and select their preferred candidate.

It stands to reason, therefore, that you could make a more *direct* hit by sending your resume directly to the specific line manager. If your resume coincides with the line manager's idea of the best candidate, it may be sent on to Personnel with a request that you be interviewed, or the manager may call you directly, depending on how formal the organization is about these things.

This does not mean you should avoid the personnel department. After all, they know about *all* of the job openings within the company, whereas a line manager may only know of those within his or her department.

You can cover both bases by following this sage advice from career columnist Joyce Lain Kennedy: "Send a cover letter and resume to *both* the manager for whom you want to work and to the personnel department employment manager." Two hits are better than one, although a direct hit to a specific hiring manager is the preferred strategy in most situations.

6. *Personalize Your Approach*

It's not enough to stuff hundreds of "perfect resumes" into envelopes, mail them to hundreds of anonymous company presidents, faceless personnel directors, numbered boxes in newspaper job advertisements, impersonal employment agencies, and unresponsive executive search firms, and then simply wait for the phone to ring. It won't happen. The truth is that the resume itself is not as important as *the way in which you use it*. The resume is a tool, nothing more.

You are much more likely to leave your imprint on the minds of prospective employers if you try to *talk* to them on the telephone *before* you send them your resume, and you are even more likely to make a strong impression if you try to talk to them face-to-face *instead* of mailing them a resume.

Jobs are not based on qualifications alone; often it's the human chemistry between the prospective employee and the employer that breaks down the barrier and brings you into the fold.

DESIGNING A STAND-OUT RESUME

Each job you apply for deserves a fresh, custom-made resume which communicates a perfect fit between your qualifications and those required to do the job at hand. There are endless ways to fashion your resume to look like it was tailor-made for the job. Here's how Tom Cotton (not his real name) designed several stand-out resumes which emphasized his most positive traits, and minimized his weaknesses.

Tom Cotton began his employment at the International Braille Press in 1980 as a collator in the shipping department. The work involved manual labor and teamwork.

A year into the job, Tom became restless. The question was, what else was he qualified to do? One day, the opportunity to run a new piece of equipment presented itself, and Tom began to alternate between that and his collating work.

Working with the plate embossing device gave Tom yet another opportunity—the chance to work closely with the main computer system. In his spare time, evenings and weekends, Tom began to study the computer manuals that were lying around the Press. Tom was in love.

People started going to Tom with questions about the computer system, and before long, Tom had worked his way into yet a third position as the part-time computer systems operator.

In 1982, Tom applied for a loan to purchase a personal computer for himself. He applied himself as zealously to this hobby as he did to his duties at work and became one of the early pioneers in the field of computer technology for the blind. He began to consult to companies that manufacture computer products for the blind and to write articles for various publications. Tom couldn't believe it, but he was becoming an expert.

By 1987, Tom grew restless again. He had spent most of his working life at the Press, and wasn't sure how or where else he could apply his skills. He wasn't even sure what his skills were, but he knew he wanted to spend *all* of his time doing what he loved most—using computer technology to make work life easier and more productive for others.

Finally, he was ready to make a move. First, he sat down and analyzed the skills that he had developed at the Press. Then, he defined two possible job objectives: teaching computer technology to beginners, or working for a local computer company that had a good reputation for hiring and promoting women, minorities, and people with disabilities. He knew himself well enough to know he could not work in an environment where "people with a difference" were not welcome.

Emphasizing his strong points, while minimizing his weaknesses, Tom designed two resumes. He used one to apply for teaching positions, and the other for computer systems work in a large corporation.

TOM COTTON
50 Winslow Lane
Belleville, MA 04706
(617) 550-8876

OBJECTIVE

A teaching position which uses my communication, diagnostic, and adaptive computer technology skills.

EXPERIENCE

1983-present: *Consultant*
¤ Analyze and make recommendations regarding product designs for adaptive technical devices for companies such as VTEK, Kurzweil Computer Products, and Votrax Speech Systems.
¤ Conducted a seminar on computer access for the blind at a rehabilitation center.
¤ Assisted in the training and configuration of a PC-based computer transcription system for a large association.
¤ Handle individual requests for computer access information over the phone, averaging two per week.
¤ Assisted in the design of a specialized driver program for braille plate embossers for a computer vendor.
¤ Published several articles on computer access technology for the blind user.

1981-present: *Systems Operator/PED Operator*
    International Braille Press, Boston, MA
¤ Provide daily user support and troubleshoot system glitches.
¤ Maintain the efficiency of IBP's computer system, including two minicomputers, various terminals, printers, software, micros, and speech output devices.
¤ Perform daily backup, create and maintain accounts, carry out file management.

102

¤ Prepare zinc plates for press, utilizing a VersaBraille as a terminal.

1980-1981: *Collator*, International Braille Press, Boston, MA
1975-1979: *Public Speaker*, United Way, New York, NY

WORKING KNOWLEDGE

Working knowledge of various hardware and software aids, including Radio Shack, Apple, and Kaypro computers, VersaBraille, Kurzweil reading machine, DECtalk, Echo Speech Synthesizer, Duxbury translation program, Enable Reader program, Braille-Edit, BETTE, BEX, and numerous terminal programs.
Proficient braille reader and cane traveler.

EDUCATION

1977: BARUCH COLLEGE, Manhattan, NY
Completed a course in FORTRAN.
1971-1974: SYRACUSE UNIVERSITY, Syracuse, NY
Persuasive Public Speaking major, candidate for B.A.

COMMUNITY ACTIVITIES

¤ Assisted in the preparation of an access guide for the handicapped for the City of Quincy.
¤ Worked as a Red Cross volunteer to coordinate communications between agency personnel and amateur radio operators assisting in local disasters.
¤ Fund raiser for a local theater group.

INTERESTS

Holder of a General Class amateur radio operator license.

References available upon request.

TOM COTTON
50 Winslow Lane
Belleville, MA 04706
(617) 550-8876

OBJECTIVE
A technical position which utilizes my computer hardware and software knowledge, as well as my ability to troubleshoot system problems, and provide a link between users and the computer system.

COMPUTER SKILLS
Hardware: Digital PDP-11/34, IBM-PC, Apple II, Kaypro 484, Radio Shack Model IV. Software: dBase II, WordPerfect, MEX, Procomm, MultiMate, QWERTY Languages: FORTRAN, BASIC

PROFESSIONAL EXPERIENCE
¤ Analyzed and made recommendations regarding computer product designs for commercial companies.
¤ Provided daily user support for key-entry operators.
¤ Dealt with system and software bugs.
¤ Maintained the efficiency of the computer system, including mainframes, terminals, printers, and micros.
¤ Performed daily backup, created and maintained accounts, carried out file management.
¤ Assisted in the design of a specialized driver program for plate embossers for a computer vendor.
¤ Configured a PC-based computer transcription system for a large association.
¤ Managed a computer-driven plate embosser for production facility.

EMPLOYMENT

1983 - present: Consultant

1981 - present: Systems Operator/PED Operator

EDUCATION

1977: BARUCH COLLEGE: Manhattan, NY
  Completed a course in FORTRAN
1971-1974: SYRACUSE UNIVERSITY: Syracuse, NY
  Public Speaking major

INTERESTS

Holder of General Class amateur radio operator license.

References Available Upon Request

§

In both cases, Tom de-emphasized his educational background, since it was clearly one of his weaknesses; mostly, he was self-taught. In fact, did you notice that Tom said he was a "candidate" for a bachelor's degree? He quit college one semester shy of completing the necessary requirements for his degree. While he didn't want to exclude the education he had obtained, he didn't want to lie, either. But he did want a chance to explain why he dropped out of school, in person, during the interview.

On the "teaching" resume, Tom stressed his personal computer skills, assuming that most beginners start with a personal computer. For the "industry" resume, he stressed his mainframe computer experience.

In one resume, he implied that he was blind by stating his braille and cane-travel skills. The particular position for which he was applying involved teaching computer access skills to visually impaired persons. In the other, he avoided the topic completely since he felt he might be screened out because of his blindness. (By the way, this turned out to be an erroneous assumption because that particular computer company had just launched a program to hire people with disabilities.)

For the teaching position, he decided a two-page resume would be best because it included information about his community activities, which he felt would emphasize his interpersonal skills. For the corporate job, he fit it into one, since he knew that computer companies receive thousands of resumes and have little time to review them in detail the first time around.

In both resumes, Tom had a clear job objective which was consistent with his qualifications. Including a job objective in one's resume is the right strategy for any job seeker who has a well-defined objective, as Tom did, and whose work history reflects the same purposefulness.

Many of us who are blind don't believe we can target our job search so specifically. As the search goes on, we tend to waver from our chosen field, hoping something—anything—will come up.

While it's true that you may start out in a less-than-hoped-for position with a promising company, you should avoid the "I'll take anything" approach. It sounds desperate, and it makes you look desperate. "Desperate" isn't a winning qualification. If you have carefully defined your job objective, you know what you want to do and you can generally communicate that feeling of confidence to others.

Knowing what you want and going after it doesn't mean you limit yourself to one job objective. Far from it. Most of us have multiple interests. Mary Tuttle, for example, has over twenty years' work experience. She has been a medical secretary at a hospital, a civil-rights investigator for the federal government, and a market support specialist for a computer company that produces products for the blind user.

In her most recent job search, she considered several possibilities, either in the civil-rights field or in market support.

To accomplish this, she designed several resumes, as Tom Cotton did, each one highlighting a different aspect of her background and targeting a different job.

If you believe that designing several different resumes is too cumbersome, think again. It's never been easier. Inexpensive word-processing technology makes this quite simple. You can number the sections in your generic resume, and use those section numbers to move text around, or delete sections altogether. For a small investment of time and money, you can produce a tailor-made resume that invites an interview.

If you don't have access to a word processor, hire a professional service. Use those section numbers to indicate to the word-processing service how each resume should be presented, depending on which job you are applying for. (Professional word-processing services can be found in the Yellow Pages under "word-processing services," "typing services," or "secretarial services.")

The key to your resume approach—indeed, the key to your job search—is, once again, to be flexible. Each job situation requires careful thought and strategic planning. There is no one right way.

Some career counselors, for example, recommend including personal information on your resume; other job counselors consider it irrelevant. The real answer is, it depends. If you are a mother of small children applying for a job as a day-care instructor, mothering is one of your skills. If you are 55 or over, experience and maturity are some of your assets. Some companies are starting to value older workers, preferring their experience and old-fashioned work values to the immaturity and more modern work ethics of younger recruits. And some companies, particularly large companies which do business with the government, want to hire people with disabilities but don't know where to find them.

The point is, use your personal data selectively and flexibly to your advantage.

USING A RESUME LETTER

Relatively few job seekers—particularly blind job seekers—can point to a steady, upward progression of responsibility within a single career. Many of us have gaps in our employment histories, either because we took time out for rehabilitation or because we have spent three or four years in a state of unemployment and progressive discouragement in the face of constant rejection from employers who discriminate. Or, perhaps, we were initially misdirected in our career goals due to insufficient counseling and support, and later found it necessary to change careers.

In this case, the traditional, chronological resume—which lists the dates of former employment and highlights career progression—would actually work to our disadvantage. The chronological resume simply would not reflect our real skills and talents.

If you fall into this category, one strategy for highlighting your abilities, rather than just your employment history, is to use the "resume letter." What makes the resume letter so attractive is that it liberates you from the well-entrenched format of the traditional resume. Now you have the freedom to present your skills, abilities, and educational qualifications in the shape and form *you* choose, within the context of a letter. Here's how it works.

The resume letter addresses the recipient by name and greets the reader with a warm, outstretched hand. It demands individual treatment. Think of how you respond to a personal letter calling you by name, compared to a computer-generated, mass-mailed letter addressed to "occupant."

In the resume letter, you describe yourself and your employment history in a more narrative style. You pinpoint how your talents and interests specifically match the job's requirements. Here is a sample resume letter:

Ms. Elizabeth Stone
Director of Sales and Marketing
Longhorn Insurance Company
10 Post Road
Boston, MA 02116

Dear Ms. Stone:

People buy products from people they like, and from companies with a strong reputation for quality and customer support. That's why I am interested in a sales training position with Longhorn Insurance Company.

Selling, as I see it, requires perseverance, a rapport with people from all walks of life, attention to detail, and honest communication. These are the skills I possess and enjoy using on the job.

I have done door-to-door selling during the summers, and have been an active recruiter of new members in a community organization. Last year I signed up more new members than any other person. Next year I plan to push that number higher.

I would like to meet you and demonstrate my "selling" skills in an interview. I will call you next week to schedule an appointment.

Sincerely,

Richard Smiles

* * * *

Using a resume letter can be risky, since it's nontraditional, so use it with discretion.

USING A FUNCTIONAL RESUME

A more common approach for people who may not benefit from the traditional chronological resume is the functional resume. It also allows you to emphasize your skills and accomplishments instead of your progressive work experience. This is particularly useful for career changers, or for people who have limited work experience.

Here is a sample functional resume. Notice how Sam's achievements are lumped into *skill areas*, rather than a chronological work history. Notice, too, how Sam stresses his *accomplishments* by using actual number and dollar amounts. He demonstrates results, not just job responsibilities.

Functional Resume

Sam Rogers
2639 South Vincent
Warrensburg, MO 64093
314-468-2393

PROGRAM DIRECTOR

Developed annual budget of over $500,000. Designed and implemented employee salary and performance review. Supervised staff. Negotiated new lease. Handled construction and decorating details in new office space and all aspects of relocation.

FUND RAISING

Developed and implemented major programs. Wrote and presented grant proposals to major corporations. Hosted corporate grant administrators. Raised a total of $550,000.

PUBLIC RELATIONS

Authored public service announcements and news releases. Appeared frequently on television and radio programs. Arranged and participated in photo sessions with public figures and media personalities. Coordinated media for major fund-raising events.

CONSULTANT

Consulted to state and federal legislators and agency directors on equal opportunity matters.

BOARD PRESIDENT

Planned and presided over board meetings and conventions. Arranged agendas, exhibits, seminars, and workshops.

CONVENTION MEETING AND PLANNING

Fifteen years' experience negotiating hotel rates and meeting and convention arrangements for groups of 10 to 3,000 on behalf of a major national organization.

1984-present: Assistant Director, ASSOCIATION FOR THE BLIND, Warrensburg, MO
1969-1983: Rehabilitation Specialist, VETERANS ADMINISTRATION, Portland, OR
1968-1969: Sales Representative, CNA, Chicago, IL
1965-1967: Instructor, Honors English, GORDON TECHNICAL HIGH SCHOOL, Chicago, IL

1965: B.A., DE PAUL UNIVERSITY, Chicago, IL

RECOMMENDED READING

There are dozens of good books on the subject of resume preparation. We have only provided an overview of some issues facing the blind job seeker.

We highly recommend Tom Jackson's *The Perfect Resume*. Jackson's book does more than just describe the process, he takes you through a full-blown career exploration *first*. The preparation of a good resume is so important that we highly suggest you bone up on the subject, beyond what we have provided here. Here are a few general tips for any job seeker:

¤ If possible, limit your resume to no more than two pages; employers are busy people.

¤ If you know exactly what you want to do, state your job objective at the top of the page. The more specific the statement is, the more you look like you know where you're going.

¤ If your career has progressed smoothly, with no discernible gaps, and if you have assumed increasing responsibility, list your past employers in reverse chronological order to indicate upward movement.

¤ Use action verbs to describe your accomplishments, *e.g.*, initiated, coordinated, operated, analyzed, evaluated, and so forth. Refer to the transferable skills listing in Chapter 2.

¤ Concentrate on results: accomplishments, problems solved, profits attained, houses built, money saved, efficiencies achieved, productivity enhanced, etc. Use hard numbers to reinforce results: number of workshops conducted, members trained, press releases written, meetings chaired, machines fixed, first-year earnings of clients placed in competitive employment, Social Security benefit dollars saved through placements, etc. Employers care more about results—what you accomplished—than they care about your job titles and dates of employment.

¤ Make absolutely certain that your resume *looks* good. A resume that is difficult to read, poorly typed, misspelled, and otherwise sloppy will project the same image about you. As a blind job seeker, you must be even more concerned about your image; most sighted people will be impressed by the fact that a blind person prepared such a flawlessly typed and attractive resume. (Quite frankly, they don't expect it.)

THE COVER LETTER: ANOTHER CHANCE TO SELL

Think about it. Before the recruiter ever gets to your resume, he or she will read your cover letter. If you have not made previous contact with this employer, the cover letter is their first impression of you. Make it a good one.

The purpose of a cover letter, like the resume letter, is to introduce yourself, personally, to the employer. In the cover letter, you have an opportunity to humanize the cold facts laid out in the resume—to put some life into them.

Unfortunately, cover letters are, for the most part, boring, boring, boring.

The worst of them start out like this: "This is in response to your advertisement of October 5th . . . for the position of . . . which was advertised in . . . ." You can only read so many openings like that before you mentally stop reading the copy. Putting a recruiter to sleep is a dangerous practice if your aim is to draw attention to yourself.

Clearly, we're not suggesting any outlandish pranks to draw the employer's attention, but we are saying that your approach should be fresh, crisp, and appealing.

Remember our friend Tom Cotton? Here is the cover letter he used, along with his resume, to eventually land a job doing exactly what he wanted to do: teaching adaptive technology to newly-hired blind employees.

Ms. Sally Ryder, Director
Job Placement, Inc.
2504 Bigelow Avenue
Willow Pine, MA 02174

Dear Ms. Ryder:

I am familiar with the excellent work done by Job Placement, Inc., in the area of employment of disabled people. Your desire to explore and offer new employment possibilities to people with disabilities is laudable.

I believe the skills, abilities, and knowledge I can offer would benefit your program and clientele. I am an excellent listener and can communicate with people on many different levels. My analytical and diagnostic skills would be valuable tools in identifying and solving problems of accommodation.

My widely varied work experience has forced me to likewise become very adaptable, often devising alternative techniques that normally would have been overlooked. My evolving technical knowledge has put me in the position of teacher to both individuals and groups as we all struggle with new adaptive aids.

Finally, I am comfortable among people of varying abilities and disabilities.

I will contact you next week to discuss this exciting position.

Sincerely,

Tom Cotton

* * * *

Notice how Tom started his cover letter by indicating his familiarity with the organization. He did his homework. Second, he moved right into a soft sell about how his specific skills would match those of the advertised position. He was direct, positive, and enthusiastic throughout. And he used his blindness as a selling point: ". . . has forced me to become very adaptable, often devising alternative techniques that normally would have been overlooked."

The agency director's name was not mentioned in the newspaper advertisement which Tom answered. Yet, his cover letter was the only one that came properly addressed to the director *by name*. Tom called the agency and found out the name of the director before sending the cover letter. His cover letter stood out from the pack, and Tom came across as a fellow who is willing to take an extra step to do a better job.

Finally, Tom said that he would contact Ms. Ryder the next week; and he did. He took the initiative.

Even though the ad asked for the applicant's salary history, Tom avoided the subject completely. Often, salary information is used by employers to screen you out, either because they can't afford you or because you earn below the market, meaning you probably can't handle this job level.

One last point. As we mentioned before, sending a resume or cover letter isn't enough. These are only the tools. YOU are the product. You must make sure that the prospective employer gets a chance to talk, and meet, with you one-on-one. A few pieces of paper cannot begin to describe who you really are.

DISCLOSURE

To Tell or Not to Tell?

Here comes the pivotal question: Should you mention your blindness in the resume or cover letter?

The arguments—both for and against disclosure—have merit. One side says "Why should I mention my blindness? If I do, they'll never call me for an interview." The other side argues

"Why should I hide my blindness? I'd rather be up-front about it."

But these are superficial arguments that don't get at the real crux of the issue. The fact is, the question of disclosure forces us to confront our own feelings about ourselves as blind people and how comfortable we are with our blindness. Many of us would like to think we are extremely confident about our blindness, that we can easily manage meeting strangers for the first time and overcome any surprise on their part. But when the real test comes—as it inevitably does in the interview—many of us simply are not so sure that we can do it after all. That realization can be devastating.

And what do the employers think? We found the employers' points of view so interesting, we decided to devote a whole chapter to them (see Chapter 5: What Do Employers Think?).

The best advice, again, is to be flexible. As each job lead comes along, evaluate which approach works best for you. Here are some factors to consider:

1. *Consider Your Personal Work History*

Many blind job seekers are simply not in a position—even if they wanted to be—to sanitize their resumes of any mention of blindness-related activities. Most blind job seekers' histories contain some experiences related to an agency for the blind, a rehabilitation facility, a residential school for the blind, or organizations of the blind. Any attempt to conceal such important facts would be quickly noticed and could work against you.

2. *Consider the Position and the Employer*

You may be applying for a position where it is a distinct advantage to mention your disability, such as a job as a braille proofreader, rehabilitation counselor, product sales representative for a computer firm that makes products for the blind, or administrator of an agency serving the blind.

Then, there is the fact that blindness is not always viewed negatively by *all* employers. There *are* companies—though you have to go hunting for them—which actually *want* to hire people with disabilities. Most of these companies simply don't know how or where to find qualified disabled applicants.

And, of course, there are those companies which, whether they want to or not, *must* hire disabled people to meet their affirmative-action goals because they do business with Uncle Sam. And don't forget about Uncle Sam himself. Both he and the state governments have, historically, led the way in hiring disadvantaged minorities.

3. *Evaluate Your Interpersonal Skills*

If you decide *not* to disclose in your resume or cover letter, you'll probably be dealing with the "shock factor." Shock is the way most employers will respond when confronted with an applicant who arrives for an interview sporting a white cane or dog. Caught completely off guard, most employers will react with silence, embarrassment, awkwardness, even hostility ("Why didn't you tell me?").

Dealing successfully with this tense situation requires strong interpersonal skills. You will be forced, in a short period of time, to put the employer at ease if you expect to get down to the business of interviewing. Which means, if you believe the axiom that *90% of the hiring decision is made in the first four minutes of the interview*, you've got fewer than five minutes to put the interviewer at ease with your blindness.

The truth is, the hiring decision is often based on a general impression of the applicant, rather than on qualifications alone. When opening the door, the interviewer wants to see an alert, self-confident person standing there, someone who has a certain seriousness but who conveys a sense of warmth and openness.

If you, on the other hand, are worried about being able to walk into the interviewer's office smoothly and quickly, worried about finding the interviewer's hand without a clumsy mishap, worried about finding the right chair to sit down in without assistance, and, at the same time, worried about putting the interviewer at ease, then you may assess the situation as "too hot to handle," preferring to reduce the stress of the "shock factor" by disclosing your blindness prior to the interview.

4. *Consider Your Values*

In weighing the pros and cons of disclosure, look deep inside at your values. You may believe that prior disclosure is an implicit acceptance of society's view that, just because you're blind, you must somehow be treated differently. You may view disclosure as a violation of your civil rights—after all, blacks and Jews aren't expected to disclose who they are (women, on the other hand, have always disclosed by the very nature of their female-sounding names).

You may feel that you have more to lose—in terms of self-respect, self-esteem, and dignity—than you have to gain by alerting the employer beforehand. You may have a profound conviction that you want to be hired on the basis of your qualifications, abilities, and desire to do the job, and that your blindness should not be allowed to interfere with those considerations. In that case, for you, the emotional cost of disclosure may be too high.

Furthermore, you may think, as one person put it, that disclosure "simply gives the employer more time to harden their already condescending and stereotyped views of blind people, and further justify their unrealistic worries over the difficulties of employing a blind person." If disclosure violates your innate sense of justice and equal treatment, then your preferred strategy may be to wait until the interview to discuss your disability.

5. *Evaluate the Process*

Since one of the best ways to garner an interview is to get a mutual acquaintance to refer you to a prospective employer,

118

this may result in automatic disclosure. It is highly unlikely that your acquaintance would call an employer and *not* mention your blindness. (In fact, you should think about how you want your mutual acquaintance to handle the subject of your blindness when they call on your behalf.)

On the other hand, if you are sending your resume to an unknown manager or personnel department, any mention of your disability may be just enough ammunition to get your resume tossed into the circular file. Remember, the tendency of most personnel departments is to look for any signs of problems in a resume.

This is perhaps the leading argument *against* prior disclosure on your resume (although this does not preclude disclosure prior to the interview). It is interesting to note, in discussions with employers, that they generally thought you should *not* disclose your blindness on your resume unless you know the company is actively recruiting people with disabilities. Neither did they recommend "the shock approach." But more on that later.

Strategies for Disclosure

If you have decided that disclosure (for a particular position) is preferable, you should next analyze the best strategy for doing so.

If you are applying for a job as a teacher at the Perkins School for the Blind, you could be direct about it and mention your blindness in the cover letter. The more difficult situation arises when you are applying for a job outside the blindness field. In that case, here are a few suggestions on where you should *not* mention it:

(a) Never mention your blindness at the top of your resume under your name and address, as some blind job seekers have done. This implies that you yourself believe that blindness is a critical factor in the employment situation.

(b) Never mention your blindness under the rubric "Health," as in "Health: Excellent, blind." This approach reinforces many employers' stereotypical assumptions that blindness and poor health are related, and confirms their unfounded fear that hiring a blind person means increased absenteeism and higher medical costs.

There are several ways to mention your blindness. If you want to introduce the subject casually, you might try this approach used by Patti Gregory when she signed up for campus interviews with law firms for a summer job:

"Openness about blindness is essential in the entire interviewing process. The resume presents a good opportunity to introduce blindness in a positive way. I listed the National Federation of the Blind as an extracurricular activity on my resume and indicated that I hold offices in the NFB as well.

"This approach proved wise for several reasons: First, it provided a starting point for discussion about my blindness. Second, this technique avoided alienating potential employers, who may feel 'fooled' or 'tricked' when a blind applicant waits until the face-to-face interview to divulge his or her blindness. Third, this approach set a healthy and positive tone for discussion early on, since it illustrated my attitudes toward blindness. Finally, by listing the NFB on my resume to indicate my blindness, I avoided overdramatization and put the issue in a proper perspective."
—from *The Braille Monitor,* June/July 1987

Some employers will not associate your activities in an organization of the blind with the fact that you are blind, so you still need to be prepared for the shock factor if you choose not to be more direct.

Another strategy—if your resume does not give any indication of your blindness and you wish to communicate this fact to the employer without triggering unwarranted concerns—is the disclosure letter. The disclosure letter works like this:

120

The Disclosure Letter

On a single page, compose a two- or three-paragraph letter to the employer in which you:

1. Disclose the fact that you are blind.
2. Describe succinctly but completely how you do, or plan to do, the job, including computer equipment, use of readers, mobility, and so forth. Convey the impression that you are flexible in your work methods, that you adapt easily to changing circumstances, and that you learn quickly.
3. Explain how well aware you are of the attitudinal barriers which, because of your blindness, may exist initially between you and your co-workers, and how you plan to help those around you feel more comfortable with your disability.
4. Mention your desire to be treated as an equal with your sighted peers and to be evaluated according to the same criteria. Describe the uncompromising rule which you always set for yourself, namely, never to trade on your blindness and use it as an excuse for not pulling your weight.
5. Mention references (not by name) who can verify that your on-the-job performance and attendance have never suffered because of your disability.

Then staple the letter to the *back* of your resume. Such a strategy is designed to achieve three important objectives.

One, by stapling the letter to the back of your resume, you can be certain that employers will read your resume without the slightest suspicion that this impressive employment and educational history belongs to a job applicant who is blind. At the very least, you will force people to focus on your job-related qualifications before their minds become clouded with concerns about your disability.

Two, by enclosing such a letter with your resume, you have come a long way toward addressing the typical employer's fears about hiring a blind person.

Three, once the prospective employer finishes reading your resume and the attached letter (which does not, by the way, take the place of your cover letter), and realizes you are blind, they may be thinking: "Well, this is an interesting approach. I'd like to meet this person." You may succeed in getting noticed and standing out from the pack.

Delaying Disclosure

You may decide not to mention your blindness in your resume or cover letter, but to wait until you get called for an interview. This strategy offers a nice compromise between not wanting to be prematurely screened out, and yet not wanting to deal with the shock factor.

If you decide on this strategy, wait until two or three days before your scheduled interview and then call and *talk to the person who will be interviewing you*. Don't leave a message with the receptionist ("Hey, Bill, you know that fellow who's coming in on Wednesday to interview for the sales position? Well, he just called to say he's blind.").

When you have the interviewer on the phone, be matter-of-fact: "I wanted to let you know, before we meet, that I am blind (visually impaired, have low vision, etc.)." Explain to the interviewer that because the number of blind people in the labor force is still very small and since most sighted people are not accustomed to seeing them at their place of work, you wanted to avoid the possibility of startling him (or her) when you walked in for the interview. On the other hand, you did not mention it before because you wanted to win the interview based on your qualifications alone.

Let the interviewer know, briefly, that you lead as full and productive a life as any sighted candidate, and that your blindness should not interfere with your ability to get the job done. Explain that you will be glad to discuss the specifics of how you will carry out your responsibilities during the interview. Add that you are looking forward to meeting him (or her).

In the chapter "What Do Employers Think?", you will see that this strategy was supported by most of the people we interviewed. They all agreed that it would be next to impossible to cancel the interview at that point, even if they wanted to, without risking a discrimination suit.

If you use this approach, however, it is imperative that you dispel from the interviewer's mind, during the phone call, any impression that you were being dishonest in not disclosing beforehand. Stress the fact that some employers (but certainly not this one) would have screened you out, based on your blindness, and that you want to be considered for the position just like anyone else.

Explain that you are now notifying the employer in order to make him or her more comfortable and relaxed in your presence. (My, aren't you thoughtful.) This is a great opportunity to make a good impression on the interviewer by handling such a tricky situation with grace and style.

If you find it too stressful to make the phone call, you could drop the interviewer a note in the mail. But this may leave the prospective employer with the impression that you yourself are uncomfortable discussing your disability, face-to-face.

Views on Disclosure

The bottom line is, disclosure is a very personal decision. There is no one right answer. To some extent, it depends on who you are, and how you view the situation.

One person may feel that, by disclosing ahead of time, he or she loses control of the way blindness will be discussed during the interview, since it gives the prospective employer more time to think about potential problems. Another person believes that by disclosing, much wasted time and effort can be avoided by not being invited for interviews with employers whose closed minds could not be changed during an interview.

It really boils down to people. Who you are and how you handle the situation, and who the employer is and how he or she handles the situation, will ultimately determine the success or failure of the interview.

Still, you can and *should* think through the issue of disclosure in each and every situation. Determining how you handle disclosure is a critical strategy which will ultimately affect your success in landing a job.

We decided, since the issue of disclosure is so controversial, to include a transcript of the discussion which took place at the employment seminar. A new paragraph indicates a change in speaker. Here's what successfully employed blind people had to say about disclosure:

§

**Employment Seminar
Discussion On Disclosure**

"If you state that you're blind on your resume, you might as well dump it in the wastebasket yourself."

"I don't think that's true."

"I don't either."

"Do you want people to know you're blind, or do you want people to know what your skills are?"

"Why make such a big deal about this? I think more people have been hurt by catching the interviewer totally by surprise. I think that does more harm than admission. If the interviewer is going to be negative about your blindness, he's going to be negative anyway."

"But there's a difference between putting it on your resume and telling them your own way."

"I think you should tell them after they call for an interview."

"Sometimes you can't avoid it. Your resume says you went to Perkins School for the Blind, or something like that. I think you should make some reference to your blindness. I think you cause yourself a great deal of harm in the interview by just walking in and the interviewer is thinking, 'Oh, my God, this person is blind! I have no idea how to deal with him (or her) or what questions to ask.'"

"You can tell him when you set up the interview."

"Right. The best time is when you set up the appointment for the interview. By that time—and it's a terrible thing to say—you've got him hooked. When he says, 'Can you come in next Tuesday?' then you tell him at that point. You say, 'I'm a blind person. Can you give me specific directions on how to get there?' It would be tough for them to say, 'Gee, Tuesday wouldn't be so good after all.'"

"I buy that. The thing I'm most worried about in their not knowing is creating a very difficult and negative situation for the interview."

"You can also put it on your resume in a positive way. I imply that I'm blind by mentioning that I use speech synthesis equipment. I also have a little blurb containing personal information, and I mention there that I'm blind but that I maintain a professional standard in spite of what is perceived as a severe handicap. It's a matter of packaging and marketing. You don't just say, 'Oh, by the way, I'm blind.' You turn it into a positive statement about yourself—you make it a selling point. You turn it around from a problem to a selling point."

"I agree with that, and I think it makes a lot of sense. What you're saying with this approach is that you have been able to overcome difficulties, and you know that's a positive thing."

"That's what employers are looking for."

"And for some people, when they see it on your resume and that you've got the guts to put it right out in front, they are kind of intrigued. 'What's this all about?'"

"But what about the person who doesn't use speech synthesis equipment, doesn't have an educational background that implies blindness; how does that person turn blindness into a positive thing?"

"He can still talk about things he's accomplished to demonstrate that he has overcome obstacles."

"In a resume?"

"Sure. We all have accomplished something, even before we got our first job, that was, quote, inspired by our blindness."

"I don't put it on my resume, but I often include it in my cover letter. Basically, I make the decision depending on the situation. Every situation is different."

"Yes, I agree. It boils down to whether it's going to be perceived as an asset. If I want a job as a disabled-student coordinator, I'm going to put it down. If I don't think it will be perceived as an asset, I don't put it down. In that case, I don't put it in my cover letter, either. I bring it up, right away, in the interview, and talk about what impact my blindness will have on the job in question. You have to decide what to do depending on the situation."

"Yes, when I applied for a job at the talking book library, I put it down because they would see it as an asset. In other cases, I played it down. Then I'd deal with it very directly in the interview. I'd say, 'Why don't you ask me some questions, even though, theoretically, the law says you can't. Let's get this blindness stuff out of the way.'"

"If you walk in and say, 'Let's get this blindness stuff out of the way,' you take the upper hand."

"That's right. You say, 'If you want to know how I'm going to do it, ask, and I'll tell you what I can and can't do. How am I going to get here? Here's how I got here today. I'm going to try to do this this way, etc. How am I going to access print? Here are a couple of ways. I've tried this device, and I have this device. How am I going to drive? Well, of course, I'm not going to drive, but here's how I'll handle that part of the job.'"

"A lot of interviewers are hesitant to confront a blind person about these issues. For one thing, it's against the law. You must take the upper hand. Bring it up right away; don't wait for the interviewer. They're sitting there thinking, 'Do I call her blind? Do I call her unsighted? Can I use words like "see" and "look"?' You know, they're still dealing with those kinds of questions. Maybe they've never met a blind person. And if they have, maybe they met someone with the typical so-called blindisms, and here they are, confronted with a person who's not like that. What do they do now? It's a totally different scene."

"But you have to be relaxed and polite about these things. Nobody's going to hire you if you make them uncomfortable."

"Exactly."

"All of this depends on how you use resumes. I tend to use them *after* the interview. They say, 'Personnel will need a resume.' You don't want to be stuck saying, 'Oh, gee, I don't have one.' I bring it with me to the interview as a backup. I don't get interviews from sending out resumes; I get interviews from personal contacts."

"In a lot of places, you have to send a resume."

"Right. So you don't always have an option. But if you do have a choice, I definitely avoid the resume until the very time I have to provide it, because I'd rather deal with the person one-on-one."

"That brings up another subject, the application form. I still don't know how to handle the question 'Is there anything you think would impede you from doing the job?' I feel you have to answer, or it sends up red flags. Do you say, 'Well, I'm blind, but I'll be able to fulfill the job requirements in spite of that,' or . . . ."

"If you feel that your blindness will not affect your ability to do the job, then I don't think you have to say anything about your blindness."

"Right. Either you can do the job or you can't."

"Well, I might believe I can do the job, but then I walk in for the interview and they see I'm blind."

"But they're asking, 'Do *you* believe it?' They're not saying, 'Do you think we believe it?'"

"This question, incidentally, used to ask, 'Do you have a physical disability?' And, of course, if you said no to that, you could be accused of lying. That's why they rephrased the question—so you can say no."

"Let's get back to the interview question, to tell or not to tell. In my own experiences, I've tried different approaches. Sometimes I simply mention special adaptive equipment on my resume, and it's implied. Other times, I didn't mention it at all and went on my skills. I just walked through the door with my white cane and the fun began. The results were mixed. Some companies were very receptive; others worried about how I would get to the bathroom. In the job I did get, I approached the company on three different levels. I came through the front door with a resume, through the side door by a personal contact, and through the back door through an employment agency. I never mentioned the fact that I'm blind. Obviously, if you use a personal contact to get an interview, they probably know you're blind. It's doubtful that a person would call up an acquaintance and refer you and not mention that you're blind. In a situation like that, I don't think you need to mention your blindness beforehand."

"What we seem to be saying is that there are times when it makes sense to put it on your resume, and times when it doesn't. But I also want to emphasize that if any of us walks into a situation where the interviewer does not know beforehand that we are blind, I don't think we should feel sorry for the interviewer. It's up to us as individuals to manage ourselves in any particular situation."

"Let me play the devil's advocate here, because I've been talking to employers—employers who have hired blind employees—and they say emphatically that they want to know before you walk through the door."

"They would probably say the same thing about blacks, but not publicly."

"No, I don't think that's it."

"Look, whether we feel bad for the employer or not, I think it's burying our heads in the sand to deny the reality that sighted people have emotional issues about blindness, and how we feel about their emotions is really irrelevant. The fact—the reality—is that they have those emotions, they have all kinds of issues, and some of them are job-related. In one interviewing process, a guy who was three levels up was asking me questions, and I was practically wetting my pants because these questions were so off-the-wall. I thought, 'If this guy's asking me questions like this, I'll never get hired.' I found out later, he was testing my reactions. He wanted to know how I would react if someone asked me off-the-wall questions about my blindness. He wanted to know if I would become hostile, or if I could be tactful and diplomatic under pressure and answer questions and be patient with other people's ignorance."

"Yes, but does he have to know about your blindness in advance in order to test your reactions?"

"I think he does. I think he has a right to have his questions ready, and to do that he has to know in advance. One day we won't have to deal with this, but we're not there yet."

"Can I say something? We all recognize that sighted interviewers have emotional problems with blindness. But what I think you were saying is that you also care about your own emotional well-being."

"That's right. I think we have the right to care about our own feelings about the process, whether to disclose or not to disclose."

"But are we trying to prove a philosophical point, or get a job? There are two sides to this issue, and I understand both of them, but I don't have a pat answer."

"I've been on the other side of the interview, when I was interviewing someone and I didn't know the person was blind. The job was for a position as a group home counselor, and I had just spent an hour with this guy, talking about his counseling experience, and just at the very end, he just laid it on me, 'Oh, by the way, I have a vision problem.' And I thought, 'Boy, this guy is the biggest turkey,' and I was more angry with him for that than any question of whether he was qualified or not."

"Well, I've had employers say to me, 'If I had known you were blind, I probably would have told you not to come in. I would have done the interview over the phone. Now that you're here, I see some of what you can do.' It's something to think about."

"We all know you're not going to get the job if you make the interviewer uncomfortable. But my argument is that if they are uncomfortable when they see you, they're going to be uncomfortable, period. I don't think telling them ahead of time will dispel their discomfort. They may act better if they have time to prepare, but that doesn't mean they'll hire you. The person who ultimately will hire you feels comfortable with you and asks questions about your blindness. If the employer doesn't ask me any questions about blindness, I know I'm not going to get the job."

"Ultimately, whether you get hired or not depends on how you and that person click. When I got hired, I did a lot of things you're not supposed to do—I had a four-page resume, which you're not supposed to do; I didn't tell them I was blind, which you're not supposed to do; I wasn't even sure I wanted the job. I got that job because the person and I got on well. My four-page resume told him I could write, and he had just hired four people who couldn't write and was very unhappy about it. I think if you're comfortable with your blindness and they're not, you're not going to resolve that in minutes."

"There's also the point that the employer would always like to know more about prospective employees; that's why they passed certain antidiscriminatory laws about ethnicity, religious affiliation, and the like. Sometimes you have to decide whether you're going to be nice to an employer and tell them how you go to the bathroom. You can't make them all happy. There's a balance there somewhere, between your own self-respect and their ignorance."

"Would you trust an employer who absolutely ignored the issue that you were blind in the interview?"

"You won't get the job."

"And what good is it if you don't get the job?"

"The point is, employers need some time to prepare for an interview when the applicant is blind. They have real questions about how your visual impairment will affect your performance on the job. It's not like they have blind people coming in once a week. They need time to prepare questions. It benefits you to have the interviewer prepared ahead of time to discuss your blindness."

"Or, volunteer the information; they don't need to ask the questions if you can give them the information they need."

"You're not giving them the information they need if you don't tell them you're blind."

"When you walk in, you are."

"Somebody once said first impressions are lasting, and that people form their first impression in the first 30 seconds of meeting someone. I think that applies whether you're blind or sighted. So you can approach this a couple of ways. You can decide that you're not going to the interview to get that particular job, you're going there to meet the interviewer and to get past their fears about your blindness. You hope that later, after you've made a good impression, maybe they'll consider you for another job."

"Maybe that would work, but I'm telling you employers feel they can't trust someone who would withhold information that *they* believe has an impact on the job. One, they feel the person has been deceitful; two, they feel perhaps the person isn't comfortable enough about their blindness to mention it up-front, and three, they feel the person is inconsiderate (a very important social flaw). It's not going to make a very good first impression. Instead of seeing, when you walk through the door, a charming, friendly, well-dressed individual, they only see your white cane or dog. If anything, you have increased what they perceive to be a high-risk situation—especially since they are not prepared to deal with it."

"I think, if you can afford to do this, you should try it both ways. Like someone said earlier, consider some of the interviews as experiences, rather than as possible jobs. Each experience teaches you something about the interview process. Let's face it, if we put it on our resume or mention it in the cover letter, the chances are, we won't be seen or considered."

"I think that's true. In fact, most employers we interviewed didn't think you should put it down on your resume, but felt you should notify the interviewer just prior to the interview."

"Letting the employer know, for me, is very upsetting. So I sort of take the middle-of-the-road approach. I use personal contacts, knowing they will mention my blindness to prospective employers. If I send my resume out for a programmer job, and it competes with others, and mine's equal or better in terms of skills, and they know I'm blind, unfortunately, I think I'd be screened out."

"I tend to agree."

"Any more comments?"

"Just one more thing. I think many people need help with an appropriate presentation of their blindness. It's a matter of packaging, and it's a skill that people need to learn." ¤

Chapter 4
Searching for the Right Job

So far, it's been easy street.

All of your activities to date—struggling with your self-assessment, your resume, and exploration of the labor market—have been *private* in nature. Coming to grips with your strengths and weaknesses, values and interests, and, of course, your attitude toward yourself as a blind person, have been kept confidential.

It's time to go public.

How different the situation feels, now that the time has come for you to pick up the telephone, hit the streets, knock on doors, and ask for permanent, full-time work. It's time to take your assessed self, with your customized resume, out to be tested—*publicly*.

Now the situation does feel threatening. Your blindness is no longer academic, and it is sure to be uppermost in the minds of prospective employers. Now the question will not be one of summer employment—when employers feel less threatened because you will only be there temporarily—but one of year-round employment. Not one of a single $2,000 payment for a two-month project, but of a continuing annual expenditure of $15,000, $25,000, or $45,000, plus benefits.

This time, the issue will not be one of temporary discomfort with the "handicap" of a blind student working alone on a sideline project, but one of concern about maintaining an ongoing relationship with a blind co-worker as a member of the team. This time, doubts will be expressed about your ability to perform; suspicions will be voiced about your effect on co-workers and work routines; and worries will surface about your overall capacity to compete on an equal footing.

It's time to get tough.

SPECIAL DEMANDS ON THE BLIND JOB SEEKER

The situation *is* different for the blind job seeker. You will need to equip yourself with the same tools sighted job seekers need, plus a few more. First, here is the standard equipment:

- A well-defined job objective
- A strong resume which relates your technical and interpersonal skills to the job
- An in-depth understanding of the world of work
- The ability to market yourself as a problem-solver to prospective employers

And, as a blind job hunter, you must also cultivate the following:

- A clear understanding of the stereotypical attitudes toward the blind you are likely to encounter in the job search process
- An unshakeable belief that, with resourcefulness and a problem-solving approach, as well as proficiency in such areas as cane travel, braille, adaptive technology, etc., you could, indeed, compete on equal terms with the sighted
- An honest desire to assist prospective employers—without anger, bitterness, or resentment—in modifying their perspective of what a blind employee can do, and to raise their expectations of your abilities

Armed with this mindset, you will have a healthy head start on the competition—sighted or blind. After all, all employers want the same thing: an employee who can do the job, lighten the work load, solve problems, remove obstacles, and smooth the path toward greater productivity.

The problem is, because of your blindness, employers often assume you will have the opposite effect. You must reverse this negative image and put your blindness in the proper perspective.

The best way to present yourself as a prospective employee who will solve, not create, problems, is to demonstrate your self-sufficiency. In your cover letter, resume, and during the interview, you will have a chance to show your strong sense of personal initiative and responsibility. Employers are going to be looking for signs that you can manage your blindness-related problems *yourself*.

If you have fallen into the dangerous habit of relying on unnecessary help from others—often extended through pity—it can have devastating repercussions on your job search, not to mention actually landing a job. You need to look closely at your own personal operating style, and, if necessary, begin to modify it toward the more independent person you would like to be—and employers want to hire.

YOUR RELATIONSHIP TO THE REHABILITATION SYSTEM

The need for you, as a blind job hunter, to demonstrate independence, self-reliance, and a sense of personal responsibility as you negotiate your way through the labor market maze also applies to your dealings with your vocational rehabilitation agency.

Many of us have grown dependent on the rehab system, and for good reasons. For one, it controls the purse strings to training in mobility, braille, and adaptive equipment. And, traditionally, the rehab system has assumed primary responsibility for job training and placement. Unfortunately, placing our futures in the hands of rehabilitation counselors—even the best rehab counselors—goes against the very qualities of self-sufficiency we should be demonstrating in the job market.

For the most part, state and private rehabilitation agencies do not enjoy excellent reputations as job placement specialists—with some exceptions, of course. Too often, counselors channel blind clients into professions deemed "suitable for a blind person," seldom exploring the full spectrum of job possibilities or assessing the blind person's real potential in the labor market.

The truth is, too many counselors do not have the requisite time to do a thorough analysis, lack career training themselves, and don't know enough about business and industry (which you may be considering) because they have not worked outside the "system," either.

All of this leads to the same conclusion: *You must assume personal control over your job-search campaign.* Does this mean you avoid the rehab agency altogether? No. It means you use the rehab agency as a resource, but you never relinquish control over the search, and the outcome, to another person or agency.

Your rehab counselor should be able to provide you with job leads, networking contacts, background information on prospective employers, occupations, and industries, and feedback on your resume, cover letter, and interviewing style. He or she can also help fund your academic studies, vocational preparation, adaptive equipment, and training in self-marketing skills.

But in the end, it's up to you to sell yourself in the labor market. After all, if you plan to work competitively but can't muster the energy or resources to find a job, how competitive will you be?

It may sound trite, but finding a job may be your first job. And this is what you want to communicate to prospective employers: that you have solved your own problem of finding the right job for you.

AN INSIDE LOOK AT
THE LABOR MARKET

Most job hunters naively think there are a fixed number of job openings, a fixed number of employees working in each organization, and a fixed number of jobs for which they could apply.

Not true. The labor market in the U.S. is constantly, and we mean *constantly*, changing. It is larger, more diverse, and more vibrant than that of any other western industrialized nation. Literally *millions of jobs change hands monthly*.

In one plant, jobs are being eliminated, while in another, or maybe in the same plant, they are being created. Some manufacturing jobs move overseas, where labor costs are lower, and the space is rented by a start-up computer company. Corporate mergers and acquisitions cause some jobs to be restructured, eliminated, and created—all at the same time.

Every day, vacancies occur when people die, retire, are sick or injured, get promoted, demoted, transferred, or fired. Some people just leave for greener pastures. People waiting to fill these slots include high school graduates, college graduates, post-graduate graduates, run-of-the-mill job hoppers, serious corporate climbers, career changers, women re-entering the labor market, minorities, people who are relocating from one state to another, or from one country or continent to another, and so on.

In such a colossal, heterogeneous, constantly changing economy, it stands to reason that *some* jobs (even a sizable number of jobs) could be found that would match your skills, interests, and values. (And we won't believe you if you say they can't.)

It also stands to reason that *some* hiring managers could be found who would be willing—in spite of your blindness—to give you a chance to demonstrate your skills and build a record of outstanding performance.

Employers come in all shapes and sizes, and they have different reasons—both good and not-so-good—for wanting to hire a disabled employee. Some want to hire disabled employees as evidence that they don't discriminate against the handicapped. Others think it's good P.R. Clearly, for some, it makes them feel good. Whatever the reason, what *you* want is a chance to prove yourself in the labor market.

So what makes the job search so difficult? Well, if the labor market were a perfectly efficient market, like a supermarket, all the buyers and sellers would come together at a single place and exchange goods. We all know it doesn't work that way. The job market is one of the least efficient markets that you'll ever encounter. On any given day, a typical job hunter has the tiniest fraction of information about possible job openings. Likewise, the employer looking for good employees is limited by the number of applicants who apply.

You might think that such a loosely structured system is greatly enhanced by the plethora of job-help services scattered across the country, such as state rehabilitation agencies, private search firms, job ads, computerized job-matching services, job fairs, student placement offices, and public employment agencies.

Think again.

According to the Department of Labor, only 20% of job openings are ever listed with employment agencies or publicly advertised. That means, obviously, that limiting your search to the want ads or employment agencies greatly diminishes your chances of finding a job.

So how are the other 80% filled? In that world you've probably heard something about: the "hidden job market."

The hidden job market is that melting pot of jobs—*millions of vacant jobs every month*—that are filled by someone who knew someone who referred or recommended them for the job. Or by someone who took the initiative to contact the employer directly. In plain English, *through personal people contacts*.

The national statistic for people with disabilities who find jobs is probably different; traditionally, people with disabilities have relied heavily on state rehabilitation agencies and other job-help services. This book supports the philosophy that today, job hunters who have physical disabilities can and should use the same techniques that have proven successful for everybody else.

WHY THE HIDDEN JOB MARKET?

A popular myth says the "best qualified" candidate always gets the job. If this were true, jobs would, theoretically, go begging *ad infinitum*.

The search for the best qualified person, presumably in the country, could mean locating, processing, screening, interviewing, referencing, and selecting indefinitely. Who says she's the best one? Maybe the next person we see will be better?

Instead, employers settle for a less draconian course of action, as follows:

1. The employer develops a profile of the *ideal* candidate, including education, training, experience, licenses, technical skills, interpersonal style, current salary level, etc.

2. Then the employer develops a profile of the *acceptable* candidate—a high school diploma instead of a college degree is okay, two years of experience instead of five would be acceptable, the salary level may be too high, compared to the salary being offered, but compensation could perhaps be adjusted.

3. Some employers carry around an image in their heads of the candidate they have in mind, which may, of course, include some illegal preferences—for instance, white, male, Protestant, tall, under 40, slim, sighted, attractive, and so forth.

Employers unconsciously tend to hire people in the image and likeness of themselves.

4. Once the qualifications have been established, the employer initiates an internal search for the candidate who meets the "acceptable" qualifications. In a large organization, the personnel department is contacted, resumes are reviewed, and employees are notified of the job opening.

5. The internal candidates who get interviewed are considered, based on the acceptable qualifications that were put down on paper—and those that were not (the image). But in the end, the candidate who gets hired will be the one who convinces the company that he or she could achieve the desired results, and whose personal chemistry caused the employer to walk away from the interview thinking "I really like this man" or "This woman would really fit in here."

In other words, the successful candidate is often the one whose personal chemistry and self-marketing strategies overpowered any shortcomings they had, in terms of qualifications, and any prejudices the employer may have had initially.

6. Only if the internal search fails to turn up a successful candidate will the search be continued outside the organization.

So, the reason 4 out of 5 job vacancies are never publicly advertised or listed, an exhaustive search for all potentially qualified candidates is never conducted, and the "ideal" qualifications become diluted as the search continues, is simply that there isn't enough time. As the old cliché goes, time is money.

IMPLICATIONS OF THE
HIDDEN JOB MARKET

Let's face it, the hidden job market means more work for you. Of course, you could get lucky. You may meet an old friend on the street or at a party who just happens to know about the ideal job for you, and they offer it to you on the spot. It could happen. It does happen.

But while luck plays a part in the job search, often what looks like luck isn't. On closer examination, you find it was "managed luck." Managed luck invariably takes place when you, the job hunter, place yourself in so many promising circumstances that "pure luck" seems to strike you.

That's what happened to Tim Reilly, who is blind. He decided on the spur of the moment to participate in a community Walk-a-Thon for charity. Although he wasn't familiar with the route, he took a chance that things would work out. Tim's attitude was "you never know who else might be there."

As luck would have it, Tim spent most of the time walking next to a broadcasting executive for a local radio station. They hit it off. In fact, they left the Walk-a-Thon a bit early to grab a bite to eat. During lunch, Tim revealed that he had often thought about a career in broadcasting, but that it seemed out of reach. At the end of the day, the executive gave Tim his card and said, "Call me."

Tim followed up on the lead and eventually got a part-time job at the station. Pure luck? It was a lucky break that Tim ended up walking next to a broadcasting executive, but it was managed luck that brought Tim to the Walk-a-Thon in the first place.

In addition to managed luck, the hidden job market means that you will have to manage your time in a highly efficient manner. Here are some helpful strategies.

ORGANIZING YOUR JOB SEARCH

1. *Set up a work space*. Organize a job-search work station for yourself in your home. Include a specific work space, typewriter, braillewriter, computer, telephone, hard files, filing cabinets, etc.

2. *Keep a regular schedule*. Dress, yes, dress for work. Be seated and ready for work at your work station at the same time every day. (And we're talking about 35-40 hours a week—the amount of time it takes the successful job hunter to find a job.)

3. *Keep an extensive filing system*. Maintain an active filing system which contains the names, addresses, and telephone numbers of prospective employers, interviewers, networking contacts, employment agency counselors, research librarians, and so forth. You will also need to organize information, such as annual reports, newspaper ads, magazine articles, convention programs, and other information. Label everything so you don't have to depend on readers or family to help you locate items when you need them.

4. *Take notes*. Always take notes following an interview or telephone conversation. Don't rely on your memory, even if you have a good one. You may think you can remember important details, but as the search goes on things will feel more and more out of control. Another important tip: Always keep some type of braille note-taking device or pocket-sized tape recorder near the phone—never keep a hot prospect waiting!

5. *Plan a week in advance*. Start small. Looking for work can seem so overwhelming that sheer fear keeps you from taking the first step. The first week, plan a strategy with goals you can meet: two cold calls and three letters. Gradually increase your quotas. You can always fill up the rest of the time with less stressful but important activities, like library research.

6. *Learn to juggle*. To effectively manage your job-search time, you'll need to keep several balls in the air at once. While your reader is tape recording some articles, start composing a letter.

While your assistant types your letter in final form, begin taking notes on the background literature she just recorded. These are the same useful skills you'll use on the job.

7. *Make every minute count.* Statistically, the more time you put in, the sooner you'll find a job. If you have just concluded an interview with one company, take advantage of the fact that you are smartly dressed to make a cold call at another company on the way home.

If you're doing library research, plan a *chunk* of time. Otherwise, no sooner have you located all the materials you need than you have to put them all back to rush out to an interview or appointment. The point is, stay active, engaged, and thinking.

JOB-SEARCH BLUES

The numbers work something like this: For every person who gets a job, 10, 50, or 200 other candidates will get a rejection letter or telephone call. Accept it; those are the odds. That's why you hear career counselors talking about the job search as "twenty-five no's followed by one yes."

Indeed, it often seems as if the whole process of finding a job were deliberately designed to inflict dejection, depression, and dismay on innocent job hunters, many of whom set out on their campaign with a bounce in their step, a note of confidence in their voice, and a presumption that the world's employers are waiting for their resume, their phone call, or their knock on the door for an interview. It just doesn't happen that way, as job hunters soon discover.

You're not alone. It's the same for all job hunters—yes, including sighted ones. Here are some job-hunting realities that make the search for work so emotionally draining:

1. The fact that 80% of all job vacancies are never publicly advertised means that you, the smart job hunter, will be compelled to work even harder to unearth them.
2. The 20% of jobs that are advertised are scattered about a highly fragmented labor market in thousands of newspapers, journals, state employment offices, private employment agencies, executive search firms, college placement offices, professional societies, job banks, job fairs, and so on. You will have to work very hard to uncover these job opportunities, too.
3. The idea of competing not only with outside job seekers but also with "insiders" who seem to have the unmistakable advantage is downright depressing.
4. The seemingly endless process of crafting, refining, and perfecting your resume to fit a particular position, and mailing it out, never to be heard from again, seems patently unfair.
5. The predicament you face, if employed, of trying to keep your job search under wraps while spending the requisite 35-40 hours a week on it (which is impossible unless you are seriously under-employed) leads you to the conclusion that your old job isn't so bad after all.
6. The need to exude a positive, can-do attitude when all you want to do is crawl into bed and pull the covers over your head consumes the rest of your energy.
7. The interminable time it takes employers to get back to you following an interview—a time, by the way, which should always be multiplied by two, no matter what the interviewer promises—leaves you feeling completely vulnerable and unable to continue prospecting.
8. The fact that when you are rejected (and the odds suggest you will be), you are rarely told the reason, and that, as a result, you take every "no" personally (rather than as a statistical norm) and begin to question your entire personhood, makes the whole process cruel and abusive.

And that's not all.

If you're blind and looking for work, the plot thickens. As difficult as the job search is for sighted job seekers, for blind job hunters it is doubly so. Not only are you faced with the same eight inhumane conditions just set forth, but you must contend with societal attitudes which typically view blind people as less competent, less productive, and more dependent than others.

Perhaps you share some of these attitudes, too. After all, you were born and raised in the same environment where these ideas were hatched. No doubt, at one time or another, you have fallen into the trap of selling yourself short—of perceiving yourself as someone less capable than you might be if you had your sight. And then there are those pesky, practical problems that really do confront you in the absence of sight. Though surmountable, they make the process even more frustrating.

Here are some additional realities that blind job seekers face:

1. Some employers—we said *some* employers—will mentally screen you out the minute they discover you are blind. They simply will not be able to consider the possibility of a blind person handling the job.
2. Some interviewers will close their eyes during the interview in a fruitless effort to imagine what it would be like to be blind. They will conclude, based on their temporary and sudden paralysis and feeling of helplessness, that you couldn't possibly manage the job.
3. Some employment agencies will be reluctant to work with you, either because they don't see blind people as viable employees or because they doubt they could find an enlightened employer who would give you a chance.
4. Some employers will make the decision to hire you, only to have second thoughts and withdraw their original offer once a problem arises, such as the late delivery of an important piece of adaptive equipment.

5. On the other side, some blind applicants—particularly those who have not had an opportunity to test their work skills—are plagued by doubts that they can compete on an equal footing.
6. Some blind job hunters are so torn by the dilemma of whether or not to disclose their blindness that the whole process bogs down.
7. Many blind job seekers find it difficult to recruit a sufficient number of readers to help them carry out the necessary background research on jobs and companies, as well as to assist them in resume and letter preparation (more on this later in the book).
8. Some blind job hunters have contacted private employers directly, only to be told, "We only work with the state vocational rehabilitation agency . . . . Why don't you go there?"
9. Some blind job seekers have sought networking contacts and have asked for referrals from relatives, friends, and neighbors, only to find, once they seriously begin to discuss jobs, that these friends and relatives don't really believe a blind person could compete equally, and avoid further contact.

You must be prepared to deal with these nine situations, and others, with effective strategies for defusing their effect on your job search.

STRATEGIES FOR SURVIVING THE JOB-SEARCH CAMPAIGN

Later, we will discuss the nitty-gritty "technical" information about how to conduct a successful job search. But first let's look at some general ways to reduce the stress associated with a typical job search.

¤ **Choose your field of interest carefully**. If you have a deep-seated attraction—a passion—for your occupation, you will be able to sustain a longer job search.

¤ **Be psychologically prepared, at the outset, for a majority of "no's" before you get to "yes!"** This is true for all job hunters, but let's face it, it's even more true for blind job seekers. The important thing is for you to believe that eventually you will receive a job offer. If you convey an attitude of "no one is going to hire me—ever," it will be picked up (and probably solidified) by the next employer you meet.

¤ **Use the experiences of your blindness to your advantage**. Focus on the assets and strengths your blindness has caused you to develop: an impressive memory for detail, organization and efficient time management, delegation and coaching in your work with readers, typists, and drivers, a method of putting people around you at ease. Or you may have a sophisticated understanding of prejudice and stereotyped thinking, which, in an increasingly diverse labor force, is a highly prized asset.

¤ **Recognize that most organizations offer many ports of entry**. If your application died in one department, push it through another one. If Personnel sits on your resume, redraft a cover letter and send it to a hiring manager in the same company. Likewise, if one hiring manager can't see the potential you offer, try another manager.

Large companies offer a multitude of choices, since they are compartmentalized into groups, divisions, departments, and sections. They may have regional offices, branch offices, plants in different states, corporate headquarters, or subsidiaries, in this country or abroad. Obviously, hitting up one manager in one department in one section of one company is just the beginning.

¤ **Don't discriminate against employers.** Remember that all sighted people aren't alike, either. If you believe you were rejected by one manager in a company because of your blindness, don't generalize to all managers in that company. To do so would be to impose the same discriminatory attitudes on all managers in Company A that you have experienced yourself, because of your blindness. People are individuals, just like you, and deserve to be treated as such.

Your task is to sift through the gamut of hiring managers whose minds are frozen by prejudice, and aim toward those with open minds, sweet reason, and a little imagination.

¤ **Companies are fluid.** If Company Z did not have a position for you in June, they may in July. Or August. We know job hunters who are afraid to contact people in companies where they were rejected 12 months earlier, fearing that the same people will be there and remember them.

This fear is based on ignorance. It is almost certain that some personnel changes took place during that time, or even that the company's attitude toward hiring people with disabilities has changed. Even if some of the same people are there, it's unlikely that they will remember you (or your resume) after several months.

¤ **Be good to yourself.** Although most career counselors advise spending 35-40 hours a week on rigorous, nonstop campaigning, only a triathlon contender could withstand such a strenuous workout. Break up your time with projects and activities that you enjoy.

¤ **Beware impending self-doubt.** There may come a time when you wonder why you kept such an upbeat attitude about the job scene. You may reach a point, as most job hunters do, of wondering why you ever saw anything positive about any aspect of your life.

Your skepticism may extend to your own feelings about blindness: Who says blindness can be managed? Maybe nursing is out of the question for a blind person, and court reporting, and stockbroking, and . . . . Maybe the interviewer was right when she said the customers might have difficulty doing business with you.

One way to beat the job-search blues is to ask for and accept support from family members and friends. Most people are sympathetic to the plight of a job seeker.

When you consider the high unemployment among the working-age blind in this country, you know it's going to be tough. But, looking at the glass half full, there are *thousands* of blind people working and performing productively. That's why it's so important to talk to successfully employed blind individuals, not only to boost your confidence, but to pick up some tactics for surviving the job-search hustle.

JOB-HUNTING RESOURCES

Use every method at your disposal in your job-search campaign. Studies show that the more avenues you try, the better your chances for success. Here are some suggestions:

I. Answering Ads

To get a good education about the state of the labor market, study ads. You can learn the latest jargon for positions (secretaries became administrative assistants), what kinds of business some companies are in (Xerox owns Kurzweil), new jobs that are being created (remember when you didn't know what a software engineer was?), and so on.

Financially secure companies generally spend more money on bigger ads than, say, small start-up companies do, especially if the position is difficult to fill. Don't be misled by the size of an ad. The bulk of new job openings in this country are being created by small businesses and nonprofit organizations.

Look beyond the obvious to the subtle implications of an ad. For example, don't ignore a large ad for highly skilled people simply because you lack those technical skills. If a large ad appears for laboratory specialists to staff a brand new facility, and you aren't a scientist, think about the other nontechnical jobs that will be created, like receptionists, office managers, bookkeepers, etc. Jumping on this tidbit of information puts you ahead of the competition.

In other words, a company may advertise IN LARGE PRINT for the most difficult jobs to fill, but not for the countless others that will also be open.

Blind ads, or ads where you are asked to respond to a nameless, faceless post office box, are a legitimate recruitment method, too. So why all the secrecy? For one thing, if the company expects a large response, they may want to shelter themselves from too many phone calls or people walking into the office to apply for the position. Or maybe they're developing a new product and they don't want the competition to know. Sometimes it's a case of not wanting the incumbent to know that they are looking for his or her replacement! Other times, the company is seeking current information on qualifications and salary scales in the general marketplace by "testing" to see who's out there and how much they cost. Blind ads should be treated in the same direct manner as open ads.

Remember that ads project the most positive aspects of any job—after all, they are selling a product, too. The wary shopper reads ads with a pinch of salt. As mentioned before, job ads may overstate the qualifications—testing the market to see what sorts of candidates are out there, and if no one responds, the ad may be rewritten with more basic qualifications. That means you should not automatically eliminate yourself from the competition simply because you don't meet a few qualifications. On the other hand, don't waste your time, and theirs, if nothing in your resume matches the job responsibilities.

You already know that only a small percentage of jobs are publicly advertised, so you should increase those odds by looking beyond your local paper. Many magazines and journals, such as *The Personnel Administrator*, focus on a particular profession and advertise those types of jobs regularly (check your local library). Often, these jobs are national in scope, which means you should be prepared to relocate. If the publication is a monthly or quarterly, that probably means the company is willing to sacrifice several months—leaving the position vacant—in order to find a truly outstanding candidate. Meanwhile, small daily papers generally contain ads on which the employer expects to move quickly, and the job could, conceivably, be filled the same day.

Some publications cater to the highly skilled, highly paid professional, like those in *The Wall Street Journal*, while other publications, such as the daily you pick up at the supermarket, may focus on lower-paying positions, like food service, janitorial, factory floor, retail sales, and so forth. Most daily newspapers run ads every day, but some, such as *The Wall Street Journal's* Tuesday edition, also publish large concentrations of jobs on a particular day of the week.

There exist publications that contain nothing but job ads. Some examples are the *National Weekly Job Report*, *Affirmative Action Register*, *Physical Therapy/Occupational Therapy Job News*, and *Opportunities in Nonprofit Organizations*.

Check out specialized publications, too. No matter what your occupation, age, religion, race, sex, geographical preference, marital status, military history, criminal record, or sexual preference, there's a publication aimed at you.

The question is, how do you manage the endless flow of information—especially if you're blind? One option, if you own a computer with a modem, is to tap into the ever-growing number of newspapers and periodicals that are online. (If you want to find out whether a particular publication is online, call the paper's office and inquire.)

If you aren't equipped technically, get a competent reader. A well-trained reader could possibly screen more ads than you could with a computer, although you sacrifice your privacy and independence. Here are a few pointers for using readers to screen ads:

¤ *Requirements for a good reader*: general intelligence, basic savvy about the world of work, some familiarity with your field of interest, a proficiency in skimming material quickly to locate specific bits of information.

¤ *Requirement for the reader's employer*: the ability to think fast and make snap decisions about whether a particular ad deserves closer examination.

¤ *Requirements for reader and employer*: the ability to communicate back and forth quickly, like this ". . . executive secretary wanted? . . . yes . . . with excellent word processing skills? . . . go on . . . and the ability to take shorthand? . . . next . . . administrative assistant wanted? . . . go on . . . with two years' experience in a marketing and sales department? . . . what salary? . . . $25,000-$30,000 . . . check it, next . . . ."

Take the time, before scanning ads, to familiarize your reader with your career objectives and work history. You don't want the *reader* to decide what you, as a blind job hunter, could do. Tell your reader you want to know about everything that meets your career goals.

Once you have identified a number of ads to which you wish to respond, follow these strategies:

1. Consider sitting on the ad for a *few* days. The sudden flood of resumes drowning the employer's desk will probably be dispensed with quickly. Surely you would prefer yours to be among the few resumes that land on the desk a little

later—after the interviewer has practically given up hope that there are any good applicants out there.

As a matter of fact, if you should come across an old newspaper ad or magazine advertisement, don't assume the position has already been filled. Even if it was filled, the hire may not have worked out. And don't believe that old, tired line, "We will keep your resume on file in case . . . ." Few people take the time to pore over old resumes that didn't make the grade the first time. So if you see an old ad that piques your interest, drop the employer a line and inquire whether, by chance, the search is still open.

2. If the ad identifies the prospective employer, your next step is to gather as much information as you can about the company, the job itself, and, if possible, the person who will make the hiring decision (remember, you have a few days to do this before sending your resume and cover letter). **If you think that doing this research is just too much work, you will probably decrease your chances of winning the interview by a factor of 10 or more.**

This research enables you to personalize your approach, to highlight the specific match between the position and what you have to offer, and to demonstrate to the prospective employer that you are a candidate who is willing to do more—in short, an outstanding candidate. The more interested you are in the position, the more research you should do. (We will discuss techniques for researching jobs later in the chapter.)

3. Next, you should *try* to identify the person who will make the hiring decision. Call the receptionist for the name of the person who heads the department where the job is located. This can be difficult, but it's worth a try. If the receptionist recognizes that your call is job-related, he or she will probably refer you to Personnel. If so, regroup and try another strategy: Call the organization's public relations department to uncover the hiring manager's identity. The point is, securing the hiring manager's name allows you to personalize your approach, and gives you another opportunity to stand out from the pack.

4. Once you have identified the hiring manager—and make sure you spell his or her name correctly—rework your resume to specifically match the job qualifications, and draft a personal letter to go with it. Don't be afraid to show some real excitement about the job. Mention that you will be calling to inquire about the position within a week.

5. *And don't forget to call within the week.* Calling the company and speaking to the hiring manager or someone in Personnel is another chance to sell your skills. It also shows you care about the job; employers like committed people.

Doing this type of homework about a position within a particular company is essential if you want to draw attention to your application. As one seminar participant put it, "Blind job seekers cannot afford to send resumes out willy-nilly into a very competitive labor market. We must do the necessary research about a particular company if we hope to get the job. We must overcome a great deal more resistance than the average job hunter, and to do that we must know how that company does business, right down to the type of office equipment they use."

II. Placing Your Own Ad

We discussed the value of placing your own ads in Chapter One. If you decide to use this strategy, here are some steps you might take:

1. *Select the Proper Targeted Audience.*

Choose the newspaper, magazine, or journal that appeals to that audience, namely, people who would be interested in your services. If you are a professional and are willing to relocate, you may select a nationally distributed professional journal; if you are a clerical worker looking for a job locally, you might advertise in a local weekly newspaper. Many metropolitan areas have weekly employment publications that list job openings in the area. *The Chicagoland Job Source* is a good example.

2. *Study the Publication.*

Buy several issues of the publication and study the ads. Study the language, format, size, and location within the publication. Then develop some thoughts about your own ad.

3. *Compose A Snappy Heading.*

A catchy heading draws the reader in—obviously, that's why newspapers and magazines hire headline writers. The purpose of a good headline is to draw attention.

Of course, mention the word "blind," and you're bound to draw attention—some positive, some not. If you think about it, though, your purpose is to attract those employers who would be open to your candidacy, employers whose imaginations are sparked by the idea of integrating a qualified blind employee into the company. Stop them dead in their tracks with headings like:

"What! A Blind Teacher?"

"I'm a Top-Notch Auto Mechanic . . . and I'm Blind"

"Blind Computer Programmer . . . ."

Try it. Don't be afraid to be daring.

III. Employment Agencies

We have a hunch that blind job seekers don't use employment agencies to the same degree their sighted counterparts do. Too bad. There are hundreds of thousands of employment agencies in existence—some good, some mediocre.

So why aren't blind job hunters motivated to use them? The explanation lies partly in the nature of the employment agency business and the incentives that drive most recruiters.

Employment agency professionals just don't sit back in their cushy offices, waiting for employers to call them with search assignments. Instead, they spend their time telephoning and personally visiting hiring managers and human resource specialists in large and small companies, trying to "sell" the special character of their agency, the depth of their candidate pool, the speed of their service, the perseverance of their counselors, and their ability to refer candidates tailored to meet individual client needs. It's dog-eat-dog in the employment agency business.

Superior employment agencies go even further by delving into the company's history, personality, philosophy, management style, organizational climate, policies and practices, as well as becoming intimately familiar with the types of people who are best suited for openings in that company. (Sounds a lot like the advice given to job seekers.)

In other words, recruiters go to considerable lengths to please their clients. Makes sense: Most of them are paid on a commission basis, and they ply their trade in for-profit enterprises. Their future relationship with a company depends on their record of successful placements.

Given this environment, agency counselors look for the best and the brightest. The game is to spend the least amount of time possible with each placement, since extra time cuts into the commission, which is fixed. That's why recruiters tend toward "safe" candidates—candidates who won't pose any potential barriers to placement. In other words, they look for people with no visible handicaps (both the physical and emotional varieties). When faced with you, a blind candidate, many counselors will:

- react negatively, seeing only the limitations you offer (your blindness) and not your strengths;

- be reluctant to invest the time and energy in you because you pose "risks;"
- be afraid of jeopardizing their relationship with employers by referring a disabled candidate.

Keep the faith. Your task in contacting employment agencies is really no different from that of contacting prospective employers: You must convince them you can do the job. You must not only overcome their initial resistance, but educate them about your skills and potential in the work force.

Scattered across the employment agency landscape are individuals who would be willing to give a qualified blind applicant a fair shot. Consider this true story, told by a seminar participant. Ken Schwartz, now working as a computer programmer for a telephone company, previously worked for a small insurance company.

"I had been with the insurance company for over three years, and during that time I started getting phone calls out of the blue from recruiters. They'd say, 'A friend of yours recommended you and speaks highly of you . . . .' I never found out who the friend was. Anyway, they'd say, 'We have a position with a good company,' and they'd throw in a buzzword or two. They'd try to get biographical information from me, because they generally didn't know that much about my background.

"At first, I just said I wasn't interested, but after three years I started to say, 'Well, maybe I'll listen. What have you got?' and then I'd mention that I'm blind. Silence. I never heard from them again. Sometimes I used that tactic just to get rid of them.

"Finally, I was really ready to make a change. I started to use a different tactic. I'd say, 'If we do this together, it's going to be a partnership. Here are the rules and here are the criteria by which I'm going to work with you. And one of them is that I'm a blind programmer with these specific skills and experiences . . . .'

"Ninety percent of them I never heard from again, until one day I found one who said, 'Okay, that's fair enough. We're going to work together; if you do this, I'll do this . . . you know, you do your job and I'll do mine.' I said, 'You get me the interview, and I'll do the rest.' That seemed like a fair swap. Whatever he did to get me the interview, I didn't care. I said, 'I want to work in these types of companies in a certain location.'

"It worked out well: He got me the interview, and I got the job. But I had to educate him about blind programmers, about myself, and really make him feel confident enough that he could go to these companies and say, 'I've got the person for you.'"

If you decide to go the employment agency route (as *one* of your job-search strategies), we suggest you *stop in* and see the first counselor who can see you. If you call ahead, you may just stir the pot about your blindness. And if you do call and don't tell them about your blindness, they may never trust you again.

Be ready to discuss your blindness honestly, and how you plan to perform certain job tasks. Your unabashed initiative (just dropping by) and obvious ability to travel independently will go a long way toward reducing their fears.

Be prepared for the worst, nonetheless. You may be the first blind person who ever set foot in the office. Some counselors may refuse to sit down with you, professing a busy day. Others may sit down with you, but only as a common courtesy and without the slightest intention of seriously considering your candidacy. Some will praise your courage (the C-word) but claim they simply don't have the professional expertise to handle "cases such as yours." Some may refer you to the local state rehab agency or society for the blind.

But sooner or later, you will meet an individual who is different. It could be a veteran counselor whose accumulated earnings are large enough for him or her to "risk" the unknown. Maybe it will be someone with a solid track record who is ready for a new challenge. Or it could be an agency

160

entrepreneur who feels a sense of social consciousness and who believes that a more enlightened approach to hiring minorities makes good business sense. Perhaps the counselor has a relative who is blind or disabled.

And consider this: Most companies today, especially the larger ones, want to demonstrate that they hire minorities (including people with disabilities). The process is made that much easier for companies when these individuals are prescreened by an employment agency. Much of the awkwardness is removed, *e.g.*, "What if I interview this disabled candidate and there isn't a match? It makes me uneasy." In this way, employment agencies are meeting the needs of their clients.

Your objective is to locate these oases of receptivity, common sense, and good will in an otherwise barren employment agency desert.

If you shudder at the thought of walking into an employment agency cold, consider this alternative: Ask the local chapter of an organization of the blind to which you belong to let you conduct a survey, under their sponsorship, of the employment agencies in your city and their policies and attitudes toward assisting disabled job seekers. The chapter's sponsorship will give the project credibility and will depersonalize the approach.

You can develop a mailing list from any of three sources: (1) the advertisements placed by employment agencies in your newspaper, (2) the Yellow Pages, (3) the membership directory of the National Association of Personnel Consultants, the principal trade association of employment agencies.

Do a professional job on the survey. Get help, if necessary. It doesn't need to be long; people are busy. Mail your survey questionnaire to the heads of these employment agencies, and enclose a brochure about the employability of blind people, with descriptive vignettes about a number of successfully employed blind individuals working in the area. Expect only a small response (the case in most survey mailings). Ask in the questionnaire if the employment agency would like to meet with a blind representative from your chapter to discuss how they might be able to better serve blind clients. Follow up any leads.

Or try this approach: Organize an educational luncheon or breakfast for area employers and owners of employment agencies, under the auspices of the local chapter of an organization of the blind. Make sure you have a good number of working blind men and women, with their supervisors, at the gathering. The best way, still, to overcome prejudice is for people to meet blind individuals who are successfully employed.

If you do succeed in finding an employment agency counselor who will work with you, make sure you check out the agency's reputation. Don't sign anything until you've had the contract checked out. Most jobs are fee-paid, and you should verify this before applying. If you don't, it could cost you plenty. Here are some ways to check out agencies:

1. Check with the Better Business Bureau. If the agency has a poor reputation, the Bureau will have a number of complaints on file.
2. Verify whether the agency is a member of the National Association of Personnel Consultants (NAPC) or of your state association of employment agencies. Membership in NAPC is conditioned upon compliance with a professional code of conduct.
3. Ask friends and business acquaintances if they know of the agency (or of any good agency).
4. Seek out the advice of corporate personnel officers.
5. Request references from individuals whom your prospective agency counselor has assisted in the past year.

If you find that the agency enjoys a fine reputation, or at least suffers no blemishes, you should still proceed with caution, as follows:

¤ Ask for a clear explanation, preferably in writing, of what services you are getting and for what period of time. Avoid non-fee-paid agencies, or, if they are, make sure you are under no financial obligation until you start work.

¤ If you are working, make sure your counselor keeps your search confidential.

¤ Resist any pressure from your counselor to accept a job that doesn't feel right to you.

¤ Consider your counselor your partner in the search. Educate your counselor about what you want (you have to know that first, of course) and what you can do. However, know that your counselor will eventually tire of your case if you, in search of the perfect job, continually turn down reasonable job offers.

IV. Executive Search Firms

The title alone, Executive Search Firm, can make you feel shy about approaching these mysterious and prestigious firms. Let's take a brief look inside.

Unlike employment agencies, executive search firms do *not* market their services to job seekers and do not solicit their patronage. They actually resist aggressive job hunters, which gives them their aloof reputation.

The reason is simple: They work exclusively for the employer. Executive search firms are retained by corporations to identify, appraise, and recommend candidates for high-level positions. Such positions rarely pay less than $60,000 a year, while the more exclusive firms wouldn't handle positions paying under $100,000. For their services, they receive 30-35% of the hired executive's first-year salary.

On the theory that "you get what you pay for," executive search firms look for men and women of superior performance, achievement, and success—people who have already established a track record and a reputation in their respective fields. So why are we mentioning these highly lucrative positions to you, the unemployed, or under-employed, or just-plain-bored job seeker who only wants a break at a medium-priced job? Because your time may come.

During the next 10 to 20 years, the employment picture for disabled job seekers should change radically as more and more employers open their eyes to their potential contributions in the labor force. As public attitudes change, more blind people will enter the labor market and eventually make their way into higher-paying and more responsible positions. If you aspire to such lofty heights, it may not be too late to begin to prepare for a brighter future. Here are some things you could do *now* to increase your potential attractiveness to executive search firms.

Since search firms look for people who are highly visible in their fields, start creating a name for yourself. Be your own PR agent. If you have some finely-tuned ideas about trends in your field, and can communicate them in writing, start by getting your name in print. Write letters to the editor of the professional journal to which you subscribe, as an opener. If Congress is contemplating some law that would have an effect on your profession, send a letter to *The New York Times* or *The Washington Post*.

Your next step might be an opinion piece to some major journal or newspaper. Many publications devote space specifically to this purpose; for example, *The Wall Street Journal features* the Manager's Journal on Mondays, and *Newsweek* magazine has the "My Turn" feature. If you want, start smaller, in your own neighborhood or suburban weekly. (Don't expect to see everything you write in print. If you do, switch to a career in writing.)

Once you've seen your name in "lights," use the momentum to get on the agenda of the next trade association conference. Or start smaller, with the local chapter meetings of your professional society. As you become better known, graduate to the overseas conferences!

Unfortunately, most of us are shy about using the word "expert" to describe our abilities. What is an expert? An expert, says Webster's II, is "a person with a high degree of skill in or knowledge of a specific subject." Experts aren't born, they're created—by you.

If you sense that an official-sounding title would give you added credibility, hold yourself out as a "consultant on . . . " and have some smart-looking stationery printed to match. Once you get an article published, hold yourself out as a "consultant and writer on . . . ," and once you have delivered a presentation at a professional society or trade association meeting, hold yourself out as a "consultant, writer, and speaker on . . . . "

Be a mover and shaker in your profession (this looks good on your resume, too). Volunteer for membership on the chapter's program committee. After a few terms in office, run for the chair. Working on the program committee gives you a great opportunity to cultivate friendships with speakers—people who generally are well connected. Schedule a program with a panel of top-notch executive recruiters. Let them see you in action as you orchestrate the program.

Once you have gained standing in the local chapter, move up to the chapter's presidency. If elected, make sure a press release goes into the newspaper. Use your office to gain greater visibility by speaking on important issues. Contact reporters who cover your field of interest, and arrange for an interview. In other words, act as your own public relations agent.

But remember: You want to project an image of *quiet* competence and *understated* elegance. A lot of bravado and exaggerated fanfare will diminish your image, rather than enhance it. When you speak, you should be confident, not combative; authoritative, not dogmatic. Corporate America still prefers the mainstream conformist personality to the outlandish maverick.

If you are active in a national organization of the blind, you undoubtedly know how the public relations game is played; use this experience to enhance your own career opportunities.

For listings of executive search firms, look at the *Directory of Executive Recruiters*, published by Consultants News, and the membership directory of the Association of Executive Search Consultants.

V. For-Profit Job-Search & Career Counseling Firms

As you skim through the paper or the Yellow Pages, you will notice ads for job search counseling firms that look a lot like employment agencies. How are they different? While employment agencies aggressively sell their services to prospective employers, job search counseling firms generally give advice and training to job *seekers* as their *raison d'être* (although some firms offer outplacement services to employers, as well).

Such organizations typically offer vocational aptitude, skills identification, and interest inventory testing. They counsel job seekers in self-assessment and career choice. Job search and career counseling firms will help you prepare your resume and cover letters, as well as decide where they should be sent. They will conduct mock interviews, sometimes with video feedback, and coach you on your weaknesses. Some firms complete the process by offering guidance negotiating salary and conditions of employment.

Sound too good to be true? Often it is. The sales strategies of these firms are, to say the least, highly seductive and extremely high-pressured. Their purpose is to dazzle you with visions of sitting back in your easy chair while they scour the labor market for the perfect job for you.

They will boast about their "comprehensive libraries of up-to-date employer directories and reference works" (the same information you could find in a good local library). They will promise to "pinpoint" prospective employers who are looking for people with your experience, skills, values, and interests. They will tempt you with claims of "professionally-crafted" resumes and cover letters (the kind which any recruiter would immediately recognize as "canned"). They will mesmerize you with "state-of-the-art video" equipment which they use during the interview skills training sessions. And they will trumpet their "over-the-shoulder" coaching in salary negotiations.

The fee for these incredible services ranges from $25 an hour on a pay-as-you-go basis to an exorbitant $8,000 up front. You should know that recently, one of the best-known career counseling firms was sued by its former clients for non-performance of services.

So, the word to the wise is, be wary. Check with the Better Business Bureau and local business licensing agencies about the firm's record of complaints, if any. Even then, proceed with caution. Think about ways in which you could get these same services for less.

For example, vocational aptitude and interest inventory tests are often administered by the career guidance centers of colleges and universities. These centers often have qualified staff who can guide you through the process of self-assessment and career choice. Main public libraries often have the same employer directories ballyhooed by these firms. You could sign up for coaching in resume preparation and interviewing skills through local classes at the YMCA, YWCA, adult education center, churches, women's groups, and community centers. The quality is often just as good, and the price is right.

If you do decide to use the services of a professional career counselor—and a good one could help you through a difficult process—ask for a written contract that spells out exactly what they will do for you, and at what price. Try to have a lawyer look it over, too.

Two books that cover the subject of career counseling in detail are *What Color Is Your Parachute?* by Richard N. Bolles (Ten Speed Press) and *Where Do I Go from Here with My Life?* by John C. Crystal and Richard N. Bolles (also by Ten Speed Press). Read them.

VI. Placement Services & Referrals through Professional Societies

Membership in a professional society is a poorly used but highly profitable job-search strategy, especially for blind job seekers. The reason we say "especially for blind job seekers" is that it offers you the chance to become known for your talents—regardless of your blindness. And some of these groups encourage the active participation of people with disabilities.

The Project on Science, Technology and Disability, of the American Association for the Advancement of Science (AAAS), was instrumental in convincing the AAAS to make its annual conventions accessible to people with disabilities. As a result of the Project's efforts, a number of other professional societies have established committees to promote greater involvement by their disabled members. It seems, however, that blind professionals have barely scratched the surface of opportunities offered through these organizations.

This is especially true in the area of placement and referral services. Here, for example, are some of the services offered to members of the American Chemical Society (ACS) by the Employment Aids Department:

Job Bank. You can submit your qualifications to a job bank, which is searched periodically on behalf of employers, on request. If your qualifications match the employer's needs, your record will be forwarded.

Chemical & Engineering News Employment Section. You can advertise your qualifications, at 55¢ per word, under "Situations Wanted."

Newspaper Employment Ad Clipping Service. ACS can send you chemicals-related employment ads clipped from 22 publications.

Confidential Employment Listing Service. You can provide ACS with a list of employers who you do *not* wish to receive your qualifications. Or you can decide what information you wish to keep confidential, like your name, your current employer, etc. If you want, you can contact the employer yourself. You receive semi-annual reports of the number of referrals made on your behalf.

National Employment Clearing House. At every ACS national meeting, a clearing house is set up for you to meet prospective employers face-to-face. Positions are posted the first day of the meeting, and interviews are scheduled.

Opportunities in Education. You can subscribe to Academic Openings, a monthly bulletin board published by ACS which specifically lists positions available in universities.

This one sampling should be enough to convince you that rich opportunities exist for job seekers who join a professional society. Most professional organizations publish membership directories—names and all—which can be used for networking in your field. The best known directory of professional societies and trade associations is the *Encyclopedia of Associations*, published by Gale Research and available in most major libraries.

VII. College Placement Services

Career planning and placement offices at colleges and universities, like anything else, come in all shapes and sizes—and attitudes. Their primary purpose is to assist graduating students in identifying, locating, and securing jobs in their fields of interest. Here are some of the services typically offered:

- Qualified psychologists who administer vocational aptitude, skills identification, and interest inventory testing
- Career counselors who offer one-on-one guidance through the career choice and decision-making process
- A well-stocked library with scads of self-help guides, directories of employers, dictionaries and encyclopedias of job descriptions, catalogues of internships, company annual reports, recruitment brochures, etc.
- Training seminars on resume writing, interviewing, networking, and so forth.
- Typing and word processing facilities
- Computerized job search programs (like SIGI+ and Discover)
- Assistance in setting up networking and informational interviews with alumni, professors, and friends of the school
- Counseling on how to negotiate pay, benefits, and working conditions
- A convenient location for interviews with prospective employers.

You would think—you would hope—that disabled students would have access to the same services as any other student. That isn't always the case. Too often, campuses segregate services by appointing a *special* career counselor for disabled students. This is done because many colleges and universities believe that students with disabilities require special services and special treatment in the job-search process because their needs are different. The truth is, the "needs" are the same—finding a good job—even though the job-search strategies may sometimes be more creative.

Working from the premise that blind students must, necessarily, deviate from the ordinary job-search path leads to discriminatory treatment—even when the intentions are otherwise honorable. The result may mean that counselors, perhaps unconsciously, direct blind students only toward those jobs that they think a blind person could do, or steer blind job applicants toward books and reading materials that only relate to blind or disabled people.

Another common practice is to encourage blind students to look for jobs only at large corporations or federal agencies, while the majority of new jobs in this country are found in small businesses.

The point is, again, that you must maintain control over your own campaign. No one should know better than you do how to conduct a job-search campaign as a blind job applicant; that is, after all, why you are reading this book.

Recognize that there are good counselors and not-so-good counselors. If you find the career placement office on your campus to be less than enlightened about your needs, consider these strategies:

1. *Get acquainted early.* Don't wait until your senior year to get acquainted; start as a freshman. Approach the placement office with your eyes open but without a chip on your shoulder. (Maybe your office is one of the good ones.) Get to know the director, as well as the staff. Let them get to know you. Let them see you as a mobile, personable, get-the-job-done kind of person.

2. *Get to know your professors.* Think of your professors and the alumni of your college as potentially your strongest allies. Most professors—particularly those in professional schools, such as business, law, engineering—have cultivated close consulting relationships with companies. Many of them have worked in

the private sector or in government service before embarking on their academic careers.

Make a point of talking to your professors about your career plans, and seeking their advice. As for your school's alumni, many of them have gone on to senior-executive levels in both the private and public sectors. Most have a "soft spot" for their alma mater and particularly for students who wish to follow in their footsteps. Some may have already signed up at the placement office as "mentors." Begin by researching the alumni directory.

3. *Take the initiative*. Don't rely on counselors to inform you of possible job openings. For one thing, they don't have the time, which is why openings are posted. Bring your own reader to skim through job ads. Get in the habit of talking to your classmates about how they stay abreast of job vacancies, internship opportunities, etc.

4. *Work in the placement office*. It's a great way to uncover job leads.

5. *Participate in campus recruiting*. Take advantage of campus recruiters who come to interview applicants. You may never again have the opportunity to schedule and talk to so many company representatives.

Be as prepared for these interviews as you would be in the employers' offices. This is a great chance to practice your interviewing skills. Learn to think on your feet in the face of difficult and unexpected questions. Start to develop a style and philosophy about how you will present and discuss your blindness.

A final note here: You should be allowed to schedule interviews the same way your sighted classmates do. If the campus counselors don't prescreen and schedule interviews for others, they shouldn't do so for you. Stay in control.

If you are no longer a student, some universities offer their placement services to alumni—even to the general public—for a fee. Check it out.

Although we have concentrated here on college-level career planning offices, the same is true for high school counseling services. Blind teenagers and their parents should know that it's never too early in a blind child's or adolescent's life to begin exploring the labor market. It's also important for your child to know that you expect them to participate in the job market—children do live up to, and even exceed, their parents' expectations.

VIII. Job Clubs and Job Fairs

Job clubs exist for job seekers to ferret out job leads together and console one another through the process of dealing with rejection. It's a support group.

Most job clubs meet on a regular basis (say, once a week), to pool information and discuss each hunter's status: "I made two cold calls which led to one interview appointment this week." Or, "I had the interview, but it was a bust." The secret of a successfully managed job club lies in the camaraderie born from the recognition that finding a job is akin to surviving boot camp.

Job clubs may be sponsored by individuals or organizations (like state employment services, rehabilitation agencies, churches, YMCAs and YWCAs, professional societies, or centers for women re-entering the labor market).

Most job clubs are free. The group leader is generally a volunteer counselor or someone who is paid by the sponsoring organization. Typically, these clubs have a "rolling" membership, which means people come and go, depending on their job status and eventual success. Sometimes the "successful" members return as volunteer or paid counselors.

To find a job club in your area, check announcements in church newsletters, neighborhood newspapers, and community bulletin boards. Advertisements of job clubs appear in *The National Business Employment Weekly*, published by Dow Jones and Company.

If you can't find a club in your area, start your own. Contact the local field representative of the Job Opportunities for the Blind Project (JOB), and see if he or she can help coordinate or lead your job support group.

Job fairs are designed to overcome some of the labor market inefficiencies described earlier. They offer one-stop-shopping opportunities for employers and applicants alike. The frequency and popularity of these fairs fluctuate, depending on the economy; they proliferate when business is booming.

Job fairs are usually organized by private employment agencies or by professional organizers. These events are held at large hotels or conference centers, which are divided into small interviewing booths. Employers participate for a fee, and the local labor market is hit with an advertising blitz just prior to the event.

Applicants take advantage of job fairs by scheduling an interview in advance or by simply walking into fairs and locating employer representatives who happen to be free for interviewing. Obviously, sending your resume to the job fair operator in advance, and pre-arranging your appointments, makes you more likely to get the interviews you want without waiting. And it makes you look organized.

Job fairs specialize, which is good for you and for employers, since the whole purpose is to pinpoint the match between prospective employers and employees. You'll see ads promoting job fairs for secretaries, for engineers, for software programmers, and so forth. In fact, you may see job fair ads welcoming people with disabilities. New York City, for example, annually sponsors a job fair under the auspices of the

Mayor's Office for the Handicapped, as does Chicago under the auspices of a group of private rehab agencies.

Here is what one seminar participant, who attended a job fair for the disabled, had to say:

"I was literally putting on my shoes, just about ready to walk out the door, when an announcement on the radio caught my attention. They were talking about the mob scene at a job fair for the disabled the previous day. Today was the last day of the fair. Luckily, I was already in a business suit (I was in a job-hunting mode). But I didn't have a truckload of resumes handy, or someone to assist me through the maze of booths at the job fair.

"I called my reader at the last minute, and she agreed to go. My next step was to get as many resumes together as I could. Thank goodness for computers and printers. By the time my reader arrived, everything was ready.

"I would like to make several points about the job fair I attended for disabled job seekers. First, I was amazed at the number of job hunters who showed up without resumes. Every employer I spoke to asked for one. *Never* forget your resume. Most employers conduct a mini-interview on the spot.

"Second, I was shocked at the lack of proper attire at the job fair. It's true, if you're applying for a job as a plumber, you don't need to dress in a three-piece business suit, but I saw plenty of people dressed for a barbecue and talking with employers about managerial positions.

"Third, and this is one of the most important points, job fairs are as crowded as Times Square on a Friday night at rush hour. You can't turn around without someone bashing your elbow. In my opinion, it is impractical to expect to maneuver through the throng without some assistance.

"Worse yet, a number of blind people were actually yelling, 'Can someone help me? Is anyone there?' It's unfair to ask other sighted, but disabled, job hunters to lend you a hand when they're job hunting, too. That doesn't mean that your assistant should accompany you right up to the booth—they should remain in the background.

"And there are other practical reasons for bringing sighted assistance to a job fair. Often, there are signs at the tables which describe the kinds of jobs those companies are recruiting for. And there are brochures about the company which can give you good insights into the firm before you actually talk to a representative about employment.

"A sighted assistant can point out those booths which are less crowded, *e.g.*, this line has fifteen people in it, while that one only has two. Plus, there are registration forms to be filled out. If you get a live prospect who says 'Here is an application form. Fill it out and return it to me before you leave today,' you must be able to do it if you want to make a good impression. I heard a blind person ask the *employer* to fill it out for him—a definite no-no.

"My final point has to do with expectations. I saw people—both blind and sighted, but mostly blind people—who were alone and uninformed about the types of jobs being offered by a rep at the booth. They proceeded to talk about jobs that were not in the arena of that company, or about jobs that were higher up the hierarchy, both monetarily and otherwise, than the candidate was qualified for. Ask questions about job openings first, before wasting people's time. Say something like 'I'm interested in accounting; what kinds of jobs are you recruiting for in that area?' Always begin by shaking hands and introducing yourself. Find out immediately about jobs that are relevant to your background.

"If you seek a management position, state it up front: 'Do you have anything in management?' The rep may respond that he doesn't, but that Ms. So-and-so back at the office might. Encourage the rep to take your resume to show to that person. If the rep seems negative, probe a little as to why. But don't waste time. If after two or three questions you find a negative attitude, thank the person and move on. Don't become a pest.

176

"Stick to questions and topics that relate specifically to the job. Don't ask about salary right away; in fact, try to avoid it altogether. Don't ask about things like how many men and women work in the office, or about how flexible the hours and benefits are. I've seen sighted and blind people do these things.

"A job fair can be successful or a real drudge. You have to keep smiling and just plow ahead. At this job fair, I got four good leads which resulted in three interviews. At another one, I got no interest at all. Who knows, someone you met that day, you might meet again in their office under different circumstances. The purpose is *exposure*. Even months later, someone may remember you because of the impression you made, even from afar."

IX. Temporary Help Agencies

Temporary help agencies do much more today than they did in the past. As labor and benefits costs go up, temporary help agencies are offering employers a better solution to their staffing needs. Some companies maintain a "permanent" temporary staff. Using temporary workers allows them to increase and decrease their workforce as their business needs change.

Temporary workers have changed, too. In the beginning, they were mostly secretaries and laborers. Today, they are nurses, accountants, engineers, data-processing specialists, construction workers, and so on.

Temporary work offers flexibility, easy labor market entry, supplemental income, and diverse work experiences. For some, temp work offers the financial means to explore other non-paying interests, like writing, painting, sculpting, and acting. It can also introduce you to a new city comfortably.

To succeed as a temporary worker, you must possess the necessary skills, be flexible and versatile, and be upbeat in your approach to people. And you must be prompt. Employers pay high hourly wages for temporary help, and their expectations are great. If you're not there on time, they won't hesitate to call the agency and replace you. It's so much easier to complain about a temporary worker.

Effective temporary workers enjoy new challenges, adapt easily to new ways of doing things, and quickly grasp new concepts. And—here's the hitch for some *blind* temporary workers—temps must be *immediately productive*. Otherwise, the expense of orientation and job accommodation outweighs the savings of hiring a temporary worker.

This is, perhaps, the strongest argument against pursuing temporary work assignments. It's too bad, too, because temporary work allows you to get an inside look at companies and jobs before you decide to take the permanent plunge.

That's not to say that because you are blind you can't pursue temporary work successfully, but it does mean you must possess a marketable skill that you can employ without considerable job accommodation. Blind people are perfectly capable of holding down temporary jobs, as long as the work methods do not have to be substantially adapted, and the blind individual can be immediately productive.

If you already know how to work various switchboards, you can be productive immediately. If you have a portable speech or braille device that enables you to handle certain jobs, you should bring it with you when you apply to the temporary agency. If you are a skilled carpenter, in the right work setting you could be productive right away.

The advantage of temporary work is the opportunity it offers employers to see you work, at first on a temporary basis, and, if you prove your effectiveness, to make you a permanent job offer. Temporary workers who make a good impression often get hired full-time when the opportunity arises.

For a listing of temporary help agencies, look at the membership directory of the National Association of Temporary Services, or study the Yellow Pages.

X. Job Opportunities for the Blind Project (JOB)

The Job Opportunities for the Blind Project is a jointly sponsored national project of the U.S. Department of Labor and the National Federation of the Blind. It is the single most comprehensive career-related program aimed at the blind job seeker. You should take full advantage of this project, not only because it works, but also because you and your family and friends, as taxpayers, have already paid for the services. Here is a sampling of what they offer:

Computerized Job Matching. At the heart of the JOB program are two computerized databases, one containing information on the qualifications, interests, and backgrounds of job candidates, and the other containing details of job vacancies from employers.

The JOB staff regularly search for matches between applicants and job openings. When a match is found, candidates are notified, and it is up to them to contact the prospective employer directly. Because the project is national in scope, the employer could be anywhere in the country.

Advice, Guidance, and Support. The project assists job seekers in improving their job-search skills. In addition to the paid staff, the project relies heavily on a grassroots network of over 100 blind volunteers scattered across the country, with a representative in every state.

Both the headquarters staff and the volunteer field representatives offer supportive guidance to any job seeker who makes use of the service. Although JOB's field representatives are not professionally-trained career counselors, they can offer what most such counselors cannot: first-hand experience with the debilitating effects of labor market discrimination on the blind job seeker. They also serve as important role models, since they have survived the labor market jungle and are gainfully employed.

Since field reps are volunteers, you should not wait for them to get in touch with you. Take the initiative and seek their advice.

The JOB Applicant Bulletin. Roughly eight times a year, all applicants registered with JOB receive a recorded bulletin comprised of three sections: (1) JOB Project news and announcements of upcoming JOB-sponsored seminars, (2) various newspaper articles on practical how-to job-search techniques, and (3) job listings from various newspapers across the country.

The idea behind the newspaper ads is not to notify candidates of possible job openings, but to acquaint labor market greenhorns with the various job possibilities in today's world of work.

Publications Aimed at the Blind Job Hunter. A real treasure chest of job-related materials in recorded and braille format is available from the JOB Project. They have occupational profiles, interviews with successfully employed blind people, skill and interest assessment guides, self-marketing and job-search campaign tips, and so on. They also have descriptions of government-sponsored programs for people with disabilities, such as the Handicapped Assistance Loan Program of the Small Business Administration and the Social Security Disability Insurance Program.

The library contains inspirational presentations about the need for blind job applicants to approach employers with "the right attitude" and a belief in their own ability to compete on an equal footing. Also available is information about employment-related technology and other job accommodations.

JOB Seminars and Workshops. Several times each year, JOB sponsors training seminars in various parts of the country. Many of these events are recorded and available from JOB.

Services to Deaf-Blind Job Seekers. The JOB Project pays attention to the needs of deaf-blind job seekers. Materials are often made available in braille.

JOB Services to Employers. The JOB Project serves employers in four distinct ways: (1) through publications that explain how blind workers can be productive employees and that help employers establish a receptive work environment, (2) through seminars for employers, designed to educate and assist them in the process, (3) by encouraging employers, on a regular basis, to send job postings to JOB, and by forwarding resumes of well-qualified JOB applicants, and (4) by responding enthusiastically to employers' requests for technical assistance in specific situations.

XI. Computerized Databases for Job Seekers

One thing computers do particularly well is transmit and store enormous amounts of information at the same time—the perfect tool for a job-search campaign.

A number of services have cropped up where employers can post positions, and applicants can post qualifications, electronically. Then each party can conduct on-line searches of the database. Here are some of the more popular computerized services:

Career Placement Registry. This computer file of eager job candidates is available to employers through the Dialog Information Services database. Candidates initiate the process by completing a data-entry or resume form and submitting it to the Career Placement Registry, with an application fee.

Employers who subscribe to the service can search the database, identify candidates, and then contact them directly. The cost for applicants is $12 for college seniors and recent graduates, and from $25-$45 for experienced candidates (the final decision is based on your current salary). This gives you exposure on the database for six months.

The Registry claims, in its promotional literature, that prospective employers conduct an average of 500 searches on the database each month and generate about 2,000 resumes. At any given time, the database contains approximately 10,000 candidate listings.

U.S. Employment Opportunities. If you subscribe to the Newsnet on-line information service, among others, you can access four separate employment-related computer files containing information on U.S. employment opportunities in banking and finance, advertising and public relations, the computer field, and the federal government. Each file has two sections.

The first section has news pertaining to that specific field, such as projections of the demand for candidates in the field, announcements of upcoming recruitment drives, predictions of layoffs, etc., and the second section contains profiles of companies in that specific field, advertisements of actual job vacancies, listings of professional associations, books, periodicals, and so forth. Files are updated every month.

All of this information is generated by Washington Research Associates, an organization that publishes the *Federal Jobs Digest* in print, as well as seventeen other similar compendia of job vacancies, each pertaining to a different occupational field.

CSI Career Network. This network is accessible to subscribers of The Source, an electronic database, and is used primarily by executive search and placement firms. It works like this. Member firms can enter information on open positions for which they are seeking candidates, as well as the qualifications of those candidates who are signed up with the agency for placement. All job vacancy and candidate listings are coded to match the particular placement firm which handles them. In that way, interested parties must contact the placement agency directly to pursue a lead.

The only way you, as an individual job seeker, can use this service is to examine the list of member firms and contact them directly. If the firm is interested in taking you on as a client, they can post your name in the file.

Online Chronicle. The Online Chronicle is available through Dialog Information Services. It covers the information industry and those professionals who work in it, like librarians, market analysts, scientific and technical researchers, etc. One of the file's components is a Jobline service containing job ads and candidate resumes. Prospective employers and job seekers submit their listings to the Online Chronicle free of charge; listings are updated every two weeks.

4-Sights Network for the Visually Impaired. This network was funded and developed specifically for the purpose of enabling blind job seekers to post their qualifications online, and for employers to post jobs and recruit disabled candidates. Unfortunately, it's off to a slow start. Currently, it contains only several dozen job vacancies and 15-20 candidate resumes.

According to the folks at 4-Sights, very few employers know about the network, most rehabilitation counselors are reluctant to share job vacancy information with fellow counselors by putting the information online, and not many blind people are using the network due to a lack of telecommunications capabilities.

Nonetheless, the network does exist, and perhaps this book will help to increase its usage. For blind job seekers living in the Michigan area, the network affords direct access to the Michigan Occupation Information System.

On-line job databases are like fickle lovers: here today, gone tomorrow. To keep abreast, you can periodically check the database directories in the reference department of your local public library. A good one is the *Directory of Online Databases,* published by Elsevier Publishing Company; another is the *Database Directory*, which can be purchased from its publisher, Knowledge Industry Publishing, or accessed electronically through BRS information technologies.

Unfortunately, by the time most of these directories are put together, they, like a lot of electronic information, are already out of date. From time to time you should also check the major electronic databases, such as Compu-Serve, The Source, Dialog, etc., to see what new on-line job databases have been hatched.

The July 1988 issue of *Online Magazine* contains an article entitled "How to Find a Job Online" which provides a detailed description of employment-related information and services that are available to job seekers by computer.

XII. Taking Advantage of "Who You Are"

As you search for work, you may be labeling yourself primarily as a *blind* job seeker. You are much more than that. You may be a Vietnam War veteran, Jewish, over 55, black, or a mother returning to work. Each of these personal traits makes you eligible for a host of job placement services designed specifically for people like you.

If you are Puerto Rican, say, you could take advantage of the National Puerto Rican Forum, which operates a job counseling and placement service for members of the Puerto Rican community. If you're an older American, there are numerous community agencies for the aging, some which are responding to growing employer interest in hiring older, more mature employees. In New York City, for example, the City Department for the Aging periodically sponsors an "Ability is Ageless" job fair exclusively for senior citizens. And the list goes on.

Try some of these avenues, too. You may be pleasantly surprised—and employed.

XIII. The State Employment Service Option

All State Employment Services are required, by law, to serve people with disabilities. There was even a time when every State Employment office was legally obliged to have at least one counselor who worked *only* with disabled candidates.

Budget cuts have eliminated that requirement—perhaps to the benefit of disabled applicants—and now all counselors work with disabled and non-disabled candidates alike.

You would be surprised at the variety of services available from the State Employment Service (although they do tend to vary from state to state).

In a typical office, those who carry the title "interviewer" get the so-called "easy" cases. If your qualifications are clear cut, your job objective well defined, and you are job-ready, you will probably see an interviewer. The interviewer will review your application form, interview you, verify your skills and interests, and refer you to appropriate employers.

If, on the other hand, you have not adequately prepared yourself for the job market—which means you didn't follow the strategies in this book—you will probably be referred to an employment counselor. Or this may happen anyway because you are viewed as a "special case." The employment counselor will work with you to clarify career goals, identify skills and interests, perfect your job-search techniques, and develop job leads.

As part of this process, the counselor may refer you to the State Employment Service's testing facility. There you may take some aptitude or vocational interest tests, or enroll in one or more training workshops in self-assessment, resume preparation, effective interviewing, targeting prospective employers, and other job-search skills.

Most people don't know that the State Employment Service system has many more job listings than typically appear in the newspaper or with private employment agencies. That's because any commercial enterprise that has federal contracts must—under a number of non-discrimination and affirmative-action statutes, including Section 503 of the Rehabilitation Act of 1973, as amended, and Section 402 of the Vietnam Era Veterans Readjustment Assistance Act of 1974—list all job vacancies with the State Employment

Service. This alone should motivate you to head on down to your local office.

All job vacancies listed with the State Employment Service are entered into a nationwide computerized job bank operated by the State Employment Service network. You can have your name and qualifications entered into the job bank for potential review by employers.

Of course, you will face the same type of situation in most State Employment offices that you do anywhere else. You may be lucky enough to get a counselor who treats you just like any other qualified candidate, or you may get someone who just can't see past your blindness. Don't sit back and wait for a tidal wave of insight to hit. Speak up and ask, politely, for another counselor. After all, State Employment offices are funded by state monies—taxpayers' monies—and you are entitled to the best possible service, just like anyone else who walks through the door.

Remember, though, that most of the staff probably have little to no experience working with a blind applicant; they will need a reasonable amount of education, from you, about what blind job applicants can do in the work force.

XIV. Working With (or Around) the Vocational Rehab System

Ah, the state rehabilitation system. What can we say that will ensure a proper perspective on a subject that evokes strong emotions among blind job seekers? First, let's say this: Although the very purpose of this book is to enable you, the blind job seeker, to go about the business of finding a job in the same manner your sighted peers do (using a few additional creative strategies to overcome a resistant market), that's not to say that you bid farewell to your state vocational rehabilitation counselor. Far from it.

Your state vocational rehabilitation agency is *charged* with several mandates that you should take advantage of, just like any other resource. These are:

1. To guide you through the career-planning and job-search process, and, in certain situations, to advocate for your interests *vis-a-vis* training facility managers, college or university administrators, and prospective employers; and
2. To finance your participation in training programs, your pursuit of college degree or vocational school certificate programs, the purchase of employment-related equipment, and the provision of many other career planning services.

There is a difference, however, between "taking advantage of" and "relinquishing control to" your state rehabilitation agency. Since most of us have grown up and lived in a home, school, even social environment where we were discouraged from taking the initiative, from venturing—both physically and emotionally—into unknown territory, and from assuming risks and responsibilities, we have allowed rehabilitation counselors to take us by the hand and tell us, chapter and verse, what we're supposed to do with the rest of our lives. We have allowed these same counselors to locate employers who are willing to consider our candidacy, and, like mother hens, lead us to the workplace or through an interview.

Moreover, since the Rehabilitation Act covers *post*-employment services, many of us have carried this dependency into the workplace itself and continue to clutch at rehab's umbilical cord throughout our working lives.

In our hearts, we know something is amiss. And yet, conditioned by years of training, we have stood on the sidelines, little more than passive observers of our own fate, paralyzed by the notion that since the agency is there to "help us," it would be inappropriate for us to complain. Or to help ourselves.

Too many years of chronic unemployment should have taught us that such a strategy is unproductive and guaranteed to keep us in a second-class status, both in the workplace and in society—a society that judges you by what work you do and how much you earn.

Too many rehabilitation counselors have fallen into the same pit, unable to distinguish between "help" that relieves a client of responsibility and "help" that encourages, even forces, the client to do more for him- or herself. The former strategy makes life easier in the short run, but fails abysmally in the long run.

We are a society founded on the principles of self-sufficiency and independence. Those lacking in these characteristics—or appearing to—will be rejected and excluded from positions of power and responsibility.

To make matters worse, most rehabilitation counselors simply are not in a position to carry out their mission effectively, because:

1. Their caseloads are so large that they cannot devote more than an average of 30 minutes per week to any individual client—not even close to the 35-40 hours a week required for an adequate job search.
2. Their performance is measured by the quantity, not the quality of cases they close, which tends to discourage time-consuming activities associated with a typical job-search and career-planning process.
3. Most counselors lack experience in the business world, and some have never worked outside the bureaucratic setting of a state rehab agency. They may lack the very skills you need: namely, the ability to interact with the business community in a professional manner.

4. A bureaucracy is a bureaucracy is a bureaucracy. In such an environment, counselors are not permitted to act freely, rapidly, and efficiently. Even the best of them—those who are creative, resourceful, and persistent—eventually tire of trying to find ways around the "system." Others never try.

As bad as the "system" is, there are ways to work with (or around) your state rehabilitation agency which will enhance your level of self-confidence, help you gain and maintain control of the process, lay the groundwork for an effective partnership with your counselor, and increase the likelihood of a successful outcome for you. Here are three strategies:

1. *Knowledge Is Power.*

At least familiarize yourself with the Rehabilitation Act of 1973, as amended, and the regulations implementing it. This is the statute that governs the operation of the federal/state rehabilitation system. Know where your agency gets its money, what services it should provide under the law, what the eligibility criteria are, and what policies your local agency has developed to carry out its mission.

Know your rights and how to appeal, if need be, to get the services to which you are entitled under the law. Find out how your agency compares to agencies in other states by networking with blind consumers in other states; this is easily done through national consumer organizations of the blind.

The more you know, the more powerful you become. To whom does your counselor report? What federal programs should be of interest to you? Among others, there is the Social Security Disability Insurance Program, the Supplemental Security Income Program, the Job Training Partnership Act, the Randolph-Sheppard Vending Facility Program, and the Javits-Wagner-O'Day Act.

The more knowledge you have, the more adept you become at "helping yourself" to the services at the rehab agency in your state.

2. *Know What You Want and What You Can Offer.*

If you really want to relinquish control to the rehabilitation system, step into the counselor's office and say, "Gee, I have absolutely no idea what I want to do with the rest of my life. I need your help badly."

How surprised can you be if your counselor promptly takes it upon him- or herself to decide *for* you? From that moment on, you are at the mercy of your counselor: He or she will enroll you in a training program, decide which college offers you the right courses, select your adaptive equipment, and, eventually, choose your employer. Only then will you realize what a huge mistake you have made.

Know what you want and what you have to offer *before* you see your counselor, or at least have some ideas. There is enough information in this book, and others, to get you to this point independently. Use the resources of the rehabilitation agency when and if *you* decide they would enhance your career search.

Tell the counselor what you want to do, and then stick to your word. If you and your counselor disagree on certain approaches, get a second opinion. Low- or no-cost aptitude testing and/or counseling can be obtained from college and university placement offices, some major public libraries, community organizations, etc. Two sources of information about such fee-paid services are The International Association of Counseling Services and the Yellow Pages of your phone book.

The bottom line is, stay in charge. Take full advantage of a system designed for your benefit by using it as a source of information and funding—not to make decisions for you. Ask your counselor to help you gather information, such as the names of blind people studying X subject in Y college, or whether a certain piece of equipment will be compatible with one that Company B uses.

When you sign your Individualized Written Rehabilitation Plan, you must have a clear idea of where you're going and how you plan to get there. You must be convinced that your choice is right, at least at this point in your life, and that you have done the necessary research, both in the library and through informational interviews, to support your goals. Many rehabilitation counselors complain that their clients have unrealistic goals and make irrational demands because they have *not done their homework*. Surely they're not talking about you!

When the time comes to actually look for a job of your choice, tell the counselor that you do not wish him or her to contact prospective employers without your *prior* knowledge. Look at it from the employers' perspective. When they hear the words "rehabilitation," "handicap," "incapacitated," "therapy," or "disability," they think **Problems**, with a capital **P**. And when you allow someone else to call for you, they think "dependent," "can't do anything by him- or herself," "needs help"—in other words, **More Problems**.

Since you will not be privy to the conversation between your counselor and the prospective employer, you have no way of knowing how you are being represented, unless you have implicit faith in your counselor. In either case, you should insist on prior notification, but feel free to give your counselor the go-ahead on a case-by-case basis. You may prefer to contact the employer yourself. Or, if the counselor has established a trusting relationship with that employer over many years, you may want your counselor to make the initial contact.

One more time, for the record: Assume personal responsibility for all decisions affecting *your* future.

3. *Be An Assertive Advocate for Yourself.*

Although there is a Biblical reference supporting the notion that the meek shall inherit the earth, the word "meek" probably did not mean "submissive," even as the slaves were being freed from Egypt.

Passivity is all too characteristic of people who have been told, from birth, to "watch out!" "take it easy!" "let me help you!" "careful!", rather than "go to it, tiger!" "go ahead, try it!" or "go on, you can do it!" Such a custodial atmosphere breeds complacency. We are taught not to disturb the status quo of the sighted world.

This is disastrous for blind job seekers trying to communicate that they can compete, and compete on an equal footing with their sighted peers. A self-effacing attitude, coupled with little or no work experience, leads to chronic unemployment.

While others, not hampered by a lifetime of diminished expectations, aggressively pursue the American dream, we are left behind, still not raising our voices, not complaining, not disturbing the status quo. Meanwhile, the status quo means 76% of us won't be working, won't be earning a living, won't be supporting our families. Obviously, we won't be inheriting the earth.

It's time for a quick course in assertiveness training. Here goes:

(a) Whenever your counselor agrees to a course of action—processing your application, enrolling you in a training program, paying your readers, arranging for a computer demonstration, getting your equipment installed, etc.—insist on a deadline, a realistic time when the task will be accomplished.

(b) If nothing has happened by the deadline, call the counselor once, twice, or three times a day (the squeaky wheel theory) until the action is completed.

(c) Keep a written record of all conversations, promises, and activities with your counselor. You may even prefer to send copies of your notes or memos to the counselor, as a written reminder.

(d) If your counselor does not return calls, does not follow through on agreed-upon activities, and, in general, just doesn't seem to be working in your best interests, begin working up the agency's hierarchy: First, contact your counselor's boss, then the district office supervisor, and on up to the agency director. Ask for a new counselor.

(e) If you do decide to file a formal complaint, be prepared for a stressful time. Moral support from others who have gone before you can be obtained from the local chapter of a national consumer organization of the blind and the Client Assistance Program, if your state has such a mechanism.

You must have detailed records on the conversations and transactions which have taken place; otherwise, your claims will be seen as more emotional than factual.

(f) Don't forget those much maligned but extremely helpful people you helped elect to office, your city council, county board, state senate or House of Representatives. One call from a congressional office to a rehabilitation agency director often is followed by a speedy resolution. But never, never abuse this alternative. Make sure your claims are legitimate before taking this action.

(g) Finally, involve the media—newspapers, radio, television—particularly their "action line" features and "letters to the editor" columns. A well-crafted, well-documented account of a qualified and willing blind candidate who did not receive adequate services from a state agency—one supported by taxpayers—could trigger action. Again, use this resource responsibly.

4. *Use Your Rehab Agency Flexibly to Your Advantage.*

As these seminar participants point out, rehabilitation agencies should not be avoided, but used as one more possible avenue to employment:

"I use the rehab agency's supportive services when I try to sell myself to a prospective employer. I say, 'There's a local agency that will help pay for equipment and training.' But I would never go to an interview with a counselor from the Commission; I go job hunting independently. But employers do like to hear that they have a fall-back agency, if they need one along the way."

* * * *

"I think it's important to use the Commission or Projects with Industry as a support service, but I would not turn over to them the responsibility for getting a job. At the request of my company, they did come in and conduct some 'sensitivity training.' None of the people I worked with had ever met a blind person. They had all the usual silly questions, and they were able to ask them of someone who would not be offended. They showed that film, 'What do you do when you meet a blind person?,' which was helpful."

* * * *

"Sometimes your rehab counselor has a relationship with an employer who is in a higher position than you might get to see just going in alone. Sometimes that's a big help . . . ."

* * * *

"You shouldn't avoid your rehab agency, because they may have relationships with important job contacts."

One final cautionary note: Some blind job hunters become so obsessed with the process of correcting what they perceive to be the grave failings of the state rehabilitation agency that they never get to the business at hand—namely, that of finding a job. Don't spend too much time on a non-productive resource.

If your state agency won't purchase a piece of equipment you need, contact the Lions or Kiwanis Clubs. If a delay in the purchase and installation of an important piece of equipment, due to the state's snail-paced bureaucracy, looks like it might jeopardize your relationship with your future boss, consider borrowing the money, paying for the equipment yourself, and settling the account with the agency when the voucher goes through.

In other words, take control.

Don't let the state agency delay you; there are often alternatives, if you take charge.

YOUR EXCUSES ARE RUNNING OUT
BY THE MINUTE

You now have 14 different avenues for exploring the open job market. *Use every one of them.* If you don't, you're not doing everything in your power to find the right job. Research shows there is a direct correlation between the number of approaches job hunters take in their search, and their eventual success.

Before you continue, however, it's time to discuss some other important tools, not only for the blind job seeker, but for the competitively employed blind worker as well. We're talking about the use of assistants to increase your productivity, both during the job search and later, on the job.

USING ASSISTANTS TO INCREASE YOUR PRODUCTIVITY

The proper use of assistants—readers, typists, drivers, and secretaries—to enhance both work-related and leisure-time productivity is poorly understood by most blind individuals. Most people use assistants sparingly, as a last resort, mainly because they fail to see their importance, and partly because good assistants are difficult to recruit.

It rarely occurs to blind people to hire typists, secretaries, or drivers **to help them increase their output many times over.** The proper use of assistants frees you from these mundane and time-consuming tasks in order to concentrate on the big picture, like strategizing, planning, and managing your job search.

Because so few blind people understand this liberating concept, many blind workers give the impression that they are slow, disorganized, and inefficient compared with their sighted co-workers. They often appear less competitive in terms of the *quantity* of work they produce, even if the *quality* is equal to or better than most. Sometimes (but not always) this is the reason blind workers find themselves isolated at work, assigned to one-person projects where they work independently and at their own pace, rather than as part of a team.

Using readers, drivers, typists, secretaries, as *tools* is simply a matter of smart time management—an extremely important factor in today's highly competitive work world. Think about it this way: Companies increase their profits by making their workers more productive, which means by increasing output within the same period of time. The efficient use of assistants can increase your productivity and make you a more desirable employee in the same way.

Some of the resistance to assistants is attitudinal. So much of life, for us, means waiting for others to do something—whether it's waiting for the taxi, the bus, braille books, special adaptive equipment, a rehabilitation counselor, and so on—that the idea of adding more "assistance" to our lives seems loathsome.

So we do without, when, in fact, recruiting, hiring, and training good assistants puts you *in charge* of your handicap, rather than allowing you to be a victim of it. It frees you from the annoying deprivation of access to the flow of information enjoyed by those around you. It frees you from dependency on an unreliable source of public transportation. Or it may free you from the anxiety of sending out typed copy if your typing skills are suspect. Readers, drivers, secretaries, and typists are tools to be used effectively. Here are some tips:

How to Find Good Assistants

Everyone you meet is a potential assistant. We say "potential" because they may not read fluently, scan efficiently, drive carefully, type accurately, or otherwise be flexible. Begin by telling your relatives, neighbors, friends, fellow students, professors, co-workers, mail carriers, vendors, doctors, etc., that you are looking for a reader. Describe the skills that a good reader possesses.

Next, prepare an announcement or advertisement stating your needs, and give it to the following organizations:

- Lions Clubs, Kiwanis Clubs, Rotary Clubs, etc.
- Churches, synagogues, mosques, temples, etc.
- Alumni associations and faculty clubs
- Women's organizations, such as the Junior League, American Association of University Women, the Business & Professional Women's Club, etc.
- Student unions, financial aid offices, fraternities and sororities (the Delta Gamma sorority considers reading to the blind their national philanthropic activity)
- Unions, professional societies, and working women's networks, such as the American Bar Association, Women in Communications, and Women in Management
- Neighborhood or city volunteer bureaus or agencies

- Corporations (many large corporations promote volunteerism among their employees) and governmental agencies
- Embassies, consulates, and emigré associations are particularly good for finding typists and readers proficient in foreign languages
- Organizations of retirees or senior citizens, such as the American Association of Retired Persons and the Telephone Pioneers of America, Area Agencies on Aging, senior housing units (where there are lots of people looking for meaningful activity)
- Public libraries (Some major city public libraries have started to organize volunteers to read to the blind. If your local library hasn't, get them started.)
- Community organizations, such as the YMCA and YWCA
- Local newspapers, where you can place an inexpensive ad
- Agencies for the blind (some already offer reader and driver assistance programs)
- College and university offices of disabled student services (although their students will receive priority, naturally)

To Pay or Not to Pay

The question "to pay or not to pay?" can't be answered with a simple "yes" or "no." The real question is, what works best for you?

If you have a paid assistant, you can expect him or her to read what you want, when you want, how you want, but that's no guarantee that they will be punctual, loyal, conscientious, or competent. Nor does paying an assistant make it any easier to fire him or her for poor performance.

Using volunteer assistants, on the other hand, has its problems, too. Volunteerism has traditionally been closely associated with "good works." It channels the charitable impulses of humankind. And that's fine. But sometimes the relationship between a volunteer reader and a blind person deteriorates to the point where the volunteer derives satisfaction and pleasure primarily from the *gratitude* of the blind individual, while the blind person, perhaps unconsciously, contributes to this by acting "needy." The relationship becomes one of subordinate (you) and superior (your volunteer reader), rather than boss (you) and subordinate (the reader).

It seems that the most successful working relationships between blind people and the people they recruit as assistants are fueled by the recognition of mutual need and satisfaction—not a relationship of "giver" and "receiver."

You may wish to pay your readers or other assistants, if you possibly can. While money does not guarantee a healthy relationship with your assistants, the act of exchanging money for service can serve as a shorthand symbol of equal status between you.

Characteristics of a Good Reader

Number one is flexibility. If you hire a competent reader who is also willing to type accurately, and drive as the need arises, you're in good shape. You also want people who:

¤ Can read straightforward literary material, as well as charts, spreadsheets, graphs, etc.
¤ Can vary the speed of their reading according to your instructions.
¤ Can rapidly locate specific spots in the text, like "the last paragraph," "the top of the second column," "the name of the manager in the last ad," etc. (This is a difficult skill to find.)
¤ Can dictate material to you, as you copy in braille, without breaks in the flow of reading.
¤ Can tape materials privately for later use, or read to you face-to-face.
¤ Can read not only at your home or workplace, but also in the library or conference hall.

¤ Can read during the day, or evenings and weekends, as required.

¤ Can respond to your reading needs in emergency situations on short notice.

You know, if you've had many readers, just how hard it is to find someone with all these qualifications—which means you should recruit a *variety* of readers, from retired people during the day, to working professionals on the weekends, and students in between.

Along with flexibility and versatility comes native intelligence—someone who can follow your instructions and someone with enough social savvy and sensitivity to understand how negative social attitudes affect blind people and how to deal with them.

Finally, you want a reader (or any assistant) to treat you as a normal, competent human being and to recognize that your blindness does not make you a more dependent person. Your reader should never take control of the reading process by deciding what to read and what to omit—that is your prerogative.

Similarly, if you hire a driver to bring you to an interview, the driver should drop you off outside the building and not presume that you need a sighted guide to escort you inside.

Screening, Training, and Motivating

Motivation works the same way for most people: If you know what is expected of you, if you possess the skills to meet these expectations, and if you are then allowed to do so—and are recognized for your efforts—you will be motivated to work hard. The same is true for your assistants.

Carefully describe the work you will assign to them and the standards against which you will measure their performance. Practice truth in advertising: If you advertise for *readers*, don't expect them to accompany you to class to take notes, or type your term paper, or drive you to the shopping mall.

Screen all potential readers carefully. Put together a reading test, or typing test, to see if they have the requisite skills. Include in the reading test an evaluation of how quickly they can respond to instructions, such as "go back two lines, please," "start that paragraph over again, please," etc.

For typists, other than speed and accuracy, you need someone meticulous in catching and correcting their own errors, and someone with impeccable taste in style and layout. After all, you will be mailing out letters and application forms to employers who will be prescreening applicants based on the appearance and presentation of the paperwork. (To evaluate their work, ask a trusted sighted friend to look it over.)

In order to give yourself and your reader a chance to work together, offer a probationary period during which you both can determine if you want to continue the working relationship.

Being a Good People Manager

Like any effective, people-oriented manager, you will need to work with your assistants, to coach them and bring them up to speed. Three critical skills that you will need are: (1) sound planning, (2) self-organization, (3) time management. The more practice you gain, the better you'll become.

Think through the agenda like this: "In preparation for my interview with Company X tomorrow morning, should I have the material about the company read by my morning reader, or should I go with my reader to the public library while it is open, and go over the company material with the evening reader?"

Here's another time-efficiency exercise: "Should I plan to work on a letter of application with my secretary face-to-face this evening, or should I compose it now and record it for her to type this evening while I go over some job ads with the reader?"

Or, "Should I print out one of my targeted resumes on my computer equipment this morning while my reader records job ads from the newspaper for me to review later, or should I work on the ads with my reader, face-to-face, and ask my secretary to print out my resume on the computer this evening?"

If you plan to work with your readers in the reference department of the library, it is *your* responsibility to familiarize yourself with what employer directories, encyclopedias, almanacs, dictionaries, and other materials are available, and where they are located. It is your responsibility to know the library's hours and where you can work, and talk, quietly. If you think and make decisions on your own behalf, others won't have to—or be tempted to.

Another serious mistake would be to relinquish all filing responsibilities to your assistant. While you may find it inefficient to label, in braille, every file in the filing cabinet, you can label every subject heading. This gives you some independent access to the information when the secretary isn't there, or when your regular reader is out sick.

Actually, you could, if you wanted to, keep track of most letters, memos, reports, brochures, bills, etc., with a little practice. Learn to identify items by the texture of the paper, the size of the sheets, the number of sheets stapled or clipped together, the type of staples used, the direction of the staples, the feel of the letterhead if raised, the way the paper is folded, the size and type of envelope used, the size and location of the stamp on the envelope, and so forth.

Some of these techniques may seem outdated and old-fashioned in an era of computers and robots. In fact, using readers, drivers, typists, and our own devices to control the flow of information has never been more important. If you expect to compete on an equal basis, you must learn to make greater and better use of these tools. You should never decline a job offer simply because you may have to "depend" on assistance. What we are striving for is psychological rather than physical independence.

It's a matter of common sense.

EXPLORING THE HIDDEN JOB MARKET

Earlier we gave you 14 places to look for employment in the open job market. But don't forget about the place where the majority of people find work: the "hidden job market."

Tapping into the "hidden job market" requires more than the usual amount of persistence, curiosity, and motivation to succeed; you'll need to assume a sort of "what the hell" attitude.

Here are the four essentials you will need to explore the hidden job market:

(1) a clear job objective,
(2) the identities of *specific* hiring managers within *specific* organizations where you would like to work,
(3) a personalized, *one-on-one* approach to targeted employers, and
(4) outstanding references.

Let's look at each essential item.

Step One:
A Clear Job Objective

We've said it before, and it's worth repeating: If you don't know where you're going, you probably won't get there. The employer is not there to solve your career-direction problems; you are there to solve the organization's employment problems. The weakest, most damaging response to an employer's inquiry about your career goals is "I'm not sure. What jobs do you have here? I'll take anything."

Pitiful.

If you want to impress hiring managers, you must succinctly and confidently express your career plans. You must know where you're going. Vague statements like "I like to work with people" or "I like working with my hands" are out. Be able to describe *where* you want to work with people, in *what* capacity, and using *which* skills.

Do you want to work with co-workers, customers, or suppliers? Is your preference indoors, outdoors, with a crew, or on your own? Would you like to work with people face-to-face, over the telephone, or through correspondence? Do you want to be serving people, counseling people, lecturing people, teaching people, or managing people? If you did your homework (see Chapter 2), you already know the answers to these important questions.

You can't find something if you don't know what you're looking for.

Step Two:
Identifying Managers and Companies

Your next task is to narrow down the list of companies where you could potentially work, and to identify hiring managers within those companies. The key is to *focus, focus, focus*.

If you are committed to a specific geographic location, or one with good public transportation, you have narrowed your scope. If you want to work for a high-tech company or an educational institution, you have focused your search a bit more. Perhaps you will target small companies, for-profit corporations, blindness agencies, social service organizations, etc. The only way to manage the overwhelming possibilities is to target your search very specifically.

But how do you find out about companies in your field of interest? There are at least three ways: (1) library research, (2) staying tuned, and (3) networking.

1. *Library Research*

Katie Boyd had been working, happily, as an instructional programmer at Contech, Inc., when—presto—a Japanese concern bought the company and laid off hundreds of workers, including Katie.

Fortunately, Katie had a clear job objective: She wanted to stay in the Chicago area, working in the field of educational programming. She began the networking process by calling her old boss and asking, "Who are our competitors in the Chicago area?" The list included 20 companies.

The process still seemed overwhelming, so Katie further refined the list by prioritizing the companies. She knew she wanted to work for a progressive, dynamic company on the move. Her first stop was the public library. She (and her reader) started with several publications, such as *The Inside Track: How to Get Into and Succeed in America's Prestige Companies*, *In Search of Excellence*, and *The 100 Best Companies to Work for in America*. She also took a look at *Rating America's Corporate Conscience*, published by the Council on Economic Priorities, which rates companies based on their social and ethical conduct.

Katie could have used other directories, such as Thomas's *Register of American Manufacturers*, *Moody's Industrial Manual*, *Martindale-Hubbell Law Directory*, *Forbes* magazine's annual listing of *The 200 Best Small Companies in America*, directories of unions, academic institutions, hospitals, government agencies, and so on. (Ask your reference librarian—now your best friend—for direction.) Several good publishers are Bob Adams, Inc., Contacts Influential, and Surrey Books, which specialize in publishing directories of major employers in particular cities.

Once Katie had prioritized her targeted companies, her next step was to *identify hiring managers within those companies*, to whom she could apply directly.

Katie's next stop was Standard and Poor's *Register of Corporations, Directors, and Executives*. S&P's *Register* is in three volumes: Volume I lists corporations, Volume II lists directors and executives by name, and Volume III is an index.

After locating the names of higher-level managers in   Volume I, Katie looked up these individuals in Volume II and found—much to her surprise—not only their names but pertinent information about their activities. For fun, she cross-referenced a few individuals in Marquis's *Who's Who in Finance and Industry*, and obtained more information, such as what degrees they held, what clubs they belonged to, what boards they sat on, even such personal information as the names of their children and wives!

Now that Katie had the names of hiring managers within certain companies in the Chicago area, she could take her research a step further. She asked the librarian to conduct an on-line computer search of the three companies that appeared at the top of her list (potentially an expensive request). She knew that in order for her introductory letter to pass the flash test, she must specifically pinpoint how her talents would match that particular company's business activities.

The librarian suggested that she refine the scope of the search. For example, did Katie want articles that appeared in newspapers, or just in journals? Would Katie prefer only those articles that related to educational software? Did she want only those citations that appeared within the last year? And so forth.

If Katie had *not* narrowed down her computer search, it might have cost her several months' pay. The library charged according to the number of citations the librarian identified for her via the computer search. Besides, Katie didn't need to know everything. She just needed to know more than her competitors did. She needed to be a little bit more prepared, a little bit more knowledgeable than her peers.

Before Katie left the library, she had one final decision to make: Did she want to pay another fee to have the library actually photocopy all of the articles that appeared in the search? No, she decided to wait and see how many citations appeared. (Another option: If Katie had a computer and a modem at home, she would have been able to access electronic databases, such as The Source and CompuServe, for some of this information. To find out if particular directories were online, she could have called the publisher of the directory. One publisher, Gale Research, is exclusively devoted to the production of directories, including *Directories in Print*.)

Once home, Katie still had more work to do on the information she had collected so far. First on the list was to verify the names she had collected, by phoning the companies. It's a good thing she did, too, because she found that one of the managers had left the company, so she quickly secured the name of her replacement by asking, "Who has taken her place? I'm planning to send some correspondence out today."

Katie not only got the new name, but she verified its spelling. Clearly, if Jan Smyth constantly received mail addressed to Jayne Smith, or, worse yet, "Dear Sir," then Katie was going to stand out in her mind as someone who cared about the really important things in life.

While Katie was on the phone with targeted companies, and before she hung up, she asked to be put through to the communications or public relations department. Once connected, she asked for copies of the company's annual report and their internal house organ or newsletter. Company newsletters are a terrific source of information about the goings-on inside a company, particularly hot new developments or new hires.

At 4:30 p.m. Katie still had a half hour to go in her "work day." She decided to take it easy, and called the National Library

Service for the Blind and Physically Handicapped (NLS) to get a copy of the Library's reference circular entitled "Magazines in Special Media."

With fifteen minutes to go, Katie asked her reader if she could treat him to a super-duper, extra large banana split—after all, they'd both had a hectic day, and knowing when to be good to ourselves (and our assistants) is part and parcel of being a good manager.

There are so many ways to research a company, and Katie used just a few of the available resources—enough, though, to get the information she needed. She could have checked such newsletter and magazine directories as R.R. Bowker's *Ulrich's International Periodicals Directory*, Oxbridge Communications' *Standard Periodical Directory*, and *Newsletters in Print,* published by Gale Research.

Many magazines and newsletters can be tapped electronically through a computer, like Newsnet, which contains some 330 professional and technical newsletters and is part of the Dialog Information Services network. Some publications are even available on computer disk.

Another good way to track companies and trends is through newspaper indexes. *The New York Times* Index, *The Washington Post* Index, *The Wall Street Journal* Index, and *The Los Angeles Times* Index, for example, are compendia of all the articles that have appeared in those newspapers, categorized by company or by individuals' names. The National Newspaper Index, produced by the Information Access Company and available on a CD-ROM, on microfilm, or online (through Dialogue Information Services), serves the same purpose. You may use these and other indexes at many public libraries.

A very simple way to identify companies in your field of interest is to check the Yellow Pages. Take advantage of this ubiquitous reference work which gets delivered to your door free of charge. If you can't coax a reader into reading the

Yellow Pages to you, call your directory assistance operator, explain that you are print-handicapped, and ask if he or she can do a little Yellow Pages research for you.

We recognize that it's difficult to gather this kind of resource information, so we've made it easier for you. Send for a copy of *The Job-Seeker's Resource Guide* from National Braille Press. Originally, we had intended to include this extensive resource directory in this book, but the information grew voluminous enough to warrant a separate publication.

2. *Staying Tuned*

You may be thinking that all this research about companies and employers seems like a lot of work. You don't know anyone else who's going to all this trouble. Maybe not. But ask yourself this: How many people do you know—how many *blind* people do you know?—who are happy with their work situations? Perhaps they don't know about the strategies in this book. Or perhaps they just don't have the motivation and energy to conduct a proper job search.

Staying tuned, keeping abreast of what's going on, puts you ahead of the competition. Look at it this way: You are an unemployed assembly-line worker. As part of your daily regimen, you have been scouring the daily newspapers. You see on the front page that Company X is opening a new plant in your area and will be using a production process you know very well. Need we say more?

You do a little research, and discover the name of the new superintendent of the plant. With very little effort, you're on your way. Instead of waiting until jobs were posted in the paper, you got a jump on the competition. Your qualifications were not buried in a sea of resumes on some recruiter's desk. In fact, you were the first person who got in to see the new super.

Or maybe you are a young, but ambitious, human resources professional whose progressive ideas about people management haven't been taken seriously by your current superiors. You read in the Who's News column of *The Wall Street Journal* that an employee relations executive whom you admire a great deal (you've been reading his ideas in various publications, and you once heard him speak at a professional society meeting) has been promoted to vice president. You drop him a line, with congratulations, suggesting a meeting when he gets settled. He's impressed with your personal note, and responds positively when you do call several weeks later.

Perhaps you've been operating a Randolph-Sheppard vending facility under the supervision of your State Agency for the Blind, but would like to leave the program and operate an independent food service business. You read a report in the Sunday paper about a survey of eating customs and habits, signaling a trend toward more take-out food. You spot an opportunity: a pizza-delivery franchise.

The point is, the future belongs to those in the know. And to those who get there first. You can be both. To keep up with today's fast-paced events, subscribe to *The New York Times Large-Type Weekly*, produced in braille by the National Library Service for the Blind and Physically Handicapped.

If your Radio Reading Service isn't reading the specific newspapers and magazines you need, call them. Tell them what your reading needs are. Familiarize yourself with the local paper first; have your reader read through all of the sections for at least a week, since many papers feature different sections on different days of the week.

The business section of the Tuesday edition of *The New York Times*, for example, carries a careers column by Elizabeth Fowler, while the business section of the Sunday edition contains a page entitled "What's New In . . . ," in which the latest trends in a particular field are reported. The Tuesday edition of *The Wall Street Journal* carries a column entitled "Labor Letter," which reports on "People and Their Jobs in Offices, Fields & Factories." Even *Women's Wear Daily* carries a thrice-weekly column called "From Where I Sit," by Samuel Feinberg, which often discusses career-related issues.

Two excellent employment columns are Joyce Lain Kennedy's, which has a question-and-answer format and appears in hundreds of newspapers around the country, and Virginia Hall's and Joyce Wessel's column, which appears in the Job Guide section of the Sunday edition of the *Atlanta Journal & Constitution*. Some of these out-of-town papers may be available at your public library or a nearby college or university.

And don't forget about audio sources of information, like TV, radio, and the recent proliferation of audio and video cassettes. You can find audio cassettes on absolutely any subject (you can even check them out, free of charge, from your local library). Call any book publisher and ask for their audio-cassette catalog. Recordings of many radio and TV programs with strong career and employment angles can be purchased after they have been aired.

Two good publications on audio resources are *The Audio Cassette Finder*, published by the National Information Center for Educational Media, or *The Video Source Book*, published by Gale Research. Both should be available at your local public library.

3. *Networking*

The value of networking has been discussed, but we want to stress the importance of using your "net" to draw in vital information from the people around you. Information resources come in human form, too. In fact, some of your best research—the most current research—will be done through people contacts.

As you research the specific companies you have identified as potential places of employment, one of the best ways to find out about the company is to get in and talk to a few employees.

Notice we did not say "and ask for a job."

"Rule Number One in the networking process," says John Erdlen, president of The Erdlen Bograd, Inc. of Wellesley, Mass., "is never make a contact and immediately ask for a job. You will inevitably be told, 'We don't have a suitable position available at this time.' The scenario will end there.

"To make the most of any contact, you should seek advice, counsel, and referrals. Naturally, the person contacted knows what the hidden agenda is—a job. But being asked for a job is a turn-off because it puts people in an awkward position. However, people will respond to a request for assistance and, almost without exception, will have other contacts in mind."

Let's review some of the principles of networking, and the reasons blind job seekers need practice using this strategy:

¤ **Good networkers are made, not born.** Networking requires initiative, motivation, and persistence. Many blind individuals haven't learned these skills. Too many people around us taught us to live cautiously, carefully, and submissively—just the opposite of the skills necessary for networking.

¤ **Networking is a "people game."** The more people you know—the more *influential* people you know—the more effectively you can play the game. Many blind people have been segregated—in schools, workshops, or at home—from the wellspring of power and powerful people.

¤ **Networking requires a free-wheeling attitude.** It's a spontaneous process of "going with the flow." We hate to beat the same drum, but these aren't the skills we were taught, right? Most of us grew up in an environment, and continue to live in a society, where restrictive do's and don'ts and prescriptive rules and regulations are a daily diet. Now we must learn the guerrilla tactics of networking. We must learn to cultivate people contacts, and to become a part of the "net." Our survival in the work force depends on it.

212

¤ **Get into the networking habit.** Everyone you meet, standing in line at the bank, on the bus, on a plane, on a boat, on a train, is a potential network contact. Get into the habit of engaging people in conversation: Ask them where they work, and how they like their work. Exchange business cards, drop them a note, follow up with a call, forward a newspaper clipping, get together for lunch, etc. The stranger you meet could be your next boss, or subordinate.

¤ **Know where to find contacts.** Much of this subject was covered in Chapter 1. Review it. And don't forget about informational interviews—a great way to network.

Good networking contacts should be able to provide you with three types of information: (a) factual information about actual job leads, the climate of the organization you are targeting, and perhaps something about the line manager you are preparing to see, (b) advice about your job-search strategy, and (c) more contacts!

¤ **Be kind to your contacts.** Contacts are to be cultivated, pampered, and *thanked*. Work around *their* schedules, and be considerate of their time. Keep your contacts informed of your progress. Provide them with useful information that you've picked up along the way. Be responsive to, not critical of, their advice. A valuable source of information will quickly dry up with too many "Oh, I've tried that and it didn't work."

¤ **Make sure your contacts represent you well.** Blind people are sometimes shocked to discover that a close personal friend, whom they have known socially for years, has expressed concern to others about their potential performance on the job, because of their blindness.

One seminar participant put it this way:

"I'm not sure blind people should use third parties in the same way sighted people do. Even people who see you as a competent person in one area may not think you are in other areas. For example, they may read for you and think you are

213

bright. But then you go out for lunch and they don't think you can handle yourself. Or it totally breaks down when you travel because they don't believe you can travel independently.

"If my brother says he's an account executive, people accept that at face value, that he can do the work. But if I say I'm an investigator, I have to explain how I do it. People automatically question whether I can do the job. You have to make sure that your 'contacts' know you well and represent you as an all-around competent person."

You now know three strategies for locating your next boss and place of employment. It requires a lot of painstaking research. Avoid this step, and you're just another fish in the sea. Master this technique, and you'll find yourself swimming among the few happily employed people you know.

Now it's time to meet your next boss.

Step Three:
Going One-On-One with Employers

How do you convince busy managers to set aside 30-60 minutes in order to get to know you face-to-face? The same way Procter and Gamble and General Mills go about selling their products: by demonstrating how their product is different from and better than the others, and through attractive packaging.

The best way to do this is to get in close. Hiring people is a risky business, and employers like to know as much as they can about potential hires before they make their hiring decision. That's why you need to get "close" and "personal."

One of the most useful and handiest tools during your job-search campaign will be your telephone. Properly used, the phone can save you time and energy, compared to the effort required to compose, type, and mail correspondence. Before you call a prospective employer, you should:

¤ Have close by whatever braille-writing, print-writing, or recording devices you use, and be ready to write. Few things are more annoying than someone who calls for information and then says, "Oh, wait a minute, I need to get something to write with."

¤ Before lifting the phone receiver, decide precisely what result you want from the call, *e.g.*, names, information, a scheduled interview, the go-ahead to send a resume, etc.

¤ Mentally rehearse the call. Decide not only what your initial question will be, but also whether you need to preface it with some kind of introductory remark. Prepare a mental guide for discussion, in case the response to your initial question is negative or not very helpful.

Chances are, your first call will be awkward. The only way to improve your phone presentation is to *practice*. Start with people who are not high on your list, or practice on a few friends. It will get easier.

We promise.

Basically, you will be making two types of calls: warm and cold. "Warm calls" are when you are telephoning a prospective employer to whom you were referred by a mutual friend. The employer is expecting your call, and will probably be receptive. Before you place a warm call, you should check with your mutual friend to make sure the referral was made. This is also a good time to find out what they said about your blindness, if anything, so you will know how to handle it over the phone.

When you make the call, refer to your mutual acquaintance, and have your agenda prepared and ready to go. Don't beat around the bush and ruin a perfectly good opportunity to make a strong impression. Keep the call short. Tell the employer that you are ready to discuss your background in detail, and ask for an interview.

Resist any request that you send your resume *before* the meeting, unless you have enough time to do the necessary job research to tailor your resume to the position. On the other hand, you don't want to appear uncooperative.

Making this kind of call, when a referral has been made on your behalf, is easier than the second type of call: a cold call. "Cold calls" are aptly named, because of the frigid response you may encounter when no one smooths the path for you. Even so, salespeople have been using the cold-call technique successfully for years, to sell their wares. So can you.

Here's how to handle it.

Call the main switchboard and ask for the name or office of the head of the organization. Relax. You won't be cold calling the CEO. It's just that the switchboard operator can't be expected to know the name and title of every specific division or department head in a large company. (The opposite is true for a small company.)

Once you have reached the secretary to the CEO, ask for the name, title, and direct extension line of the manager you are trying to contact. For example, "Could you please tell me who is in charge of your marketing and sales department?" "What is his or her exact title?" "Could you please give me the direct extension?"

If the secretary should spout forth the nine-nastiest-words-in-telephone-history, "What, may I ask, is this in reference to?", simply respond, "It's a business-related matter." If pressed further, answer that you are conducting some research on the company. Be pleasant, but persistent.

An alternative to calling the office of the CEO would be to call the organization's public relations department or office of public information.

Once you have the person's "vitals," hang up and call the extension—not to talk to the person, but to verify the information. You are not yet ready to speak to your party. First you must research the person and the company, as discussed previously. And don't forget to call Public Relations and ask for a copy of the annual report and company newsletter.

After you have conducted the research, you're ready to call the targeted hiring manager. Again, rehearse your telephone presentation, including what you will say to the secretary who answers the phone. Think through all the possible responses, and decide how you will react. Practice a few cold calls with friends. Record the conversations, and play them back. (Now, aren't you glad you didn't say *that* to your future boss?)

The calls will get easier the more you practice, but isn't that true about most things? Develop a concise and persuasive self-marketing presentation, which should last no longer than 90 *seconds*. First, say what motivated you to call in the first place (this could be an article you read, some first-hand experience with the company's products, a new product release that interests you, etc.). Then cover your current career objective and work status, your professional experience, your skills, your interests, and most important of all, your potential value to the organization.

But don't hang up yet. Don't get off the phone until you have *asked* for an interview. Every good salesperson knows you must ask for the order, no matter how persuasive your presentation. If you want to mention your blindness here, do so. If the manager responds that there are no job openings, ask if you can have a 15-20 minute informal meeting to discuss other possible career opportunities in the industry. Argue that you would like to get a closer look at the company. Be gently assertive. Remember, everything you say, and every way you say it, is creating an image in the hiring manager's mind about who you are. Make it positive.

Be aware that you may never get through the secretary to the hiring manager. The typical responses are "She's away from her desk," "He's out of the office," ". . . at lunch," ". . . on the other line," and so on. Try a few more times before giving up.

217

Then try these strategies for getting around the secretary problem.

Preferably, call before 9:00 a.m. or after 5:00 p.m.; conscientious managers are often in the office before their secretaries, and after. Or try calling during the lunch hour, when the manager may be answering calls personally. You could even try the office on weekends.

There are some risks to this approach, says John Erdlen of The Erdlen Bograd Group, Inc. "If a person is working at this time, your interruptions could be more aggravating than normal." Proceed with caution.

If you do get through to the hiring manager, don't be a time hog. Show that you are conscious of time by saying that you will take just two minutes of his or her time—and stick to it. The manager may prefer to call you back at a more opportune time. Accept gladly, and don't forget to leave your answering machine on when you go out. (Avoid cutesy or comical messages with a musical or raucous background.)

Cold calling can be hard on the ego. It's loaded with rejection. You can't take it personally. No salesperson who does lasts very long in the business. Sometimes it will simply be the case that there are no job openings. This happens during periods of economic recession, corporate downsizing, and across-the-board job freezes. Other times, the lack of job vacancies is a short-term situation; staffing requirements change from one day or week to the next. Sometimes vacancies are available but they don't match your skills and interests. And, of course, sometimes you will be rejected because your presentation was not good enough, at least not in the mind of the prospective employer.

Keep your antennae up. If your request for an interview is rejected, try to find out why. If you get the feeling that the lack of job openings is temporary, wait two or three months and call again. If you think your qualifications were a factor, ask the manager candidly in what way your skills may be lacking, and what she or he suggests you could do to improve them. Finally, if you have absolutely no idea why you were denied an interview, ask the manager for tips on how you could improve your presentation.

Very often, your request for an interview will be rejected but you will be asked to send a resume. Consider this an accomplishment. Your phone presentation was savvy enough to convince this prospective employer that he or she should take a look at your qualifications. Thank the manager for speaking with you.

Seize this opportunity to enhance your image by reworking your resume and cover letter to fit more closely the overall requirements of the position. When the manager receives your letter, your name will be familiar and your targeted resume and cover letter will strengthen the impression you made over the phone. Wait four or five days and call again to make sure your materials were received.

If after two weeks you still have not heard back from the prospective employer (and this is entirely likely), call again and express your interest. Be careful not to make a pest of yourself, but be persistent about your interest in the job and the company.

Going one-on-one with prospective employers should result in several interviews. If not, review your approach and ask for some assistance from a career counselor. Your task, here, is to contact enough hiring managers to increase your odds of being invited for an interview. Getting the interview is your goal. Once you have secured an interview appointment, you must prepare the fourth item: outstanding references.

**Step Four:
Acquiring Outstanding References**

References are people who will vouch for your technical qualifications and interpersonal skills to a prospective employer. You need to ask your references for permission to use their names and to give out their phone numbers to prospective employers. You want to do this before you start interviewing; you may need to supply references during the first interview.

Start by contacting your references, preferably by phone, and explaining that you are conducting a job search. Briefly discuss the types of jobs you are searching for, and any potential leads you are pursuing. If you have a specific job in mind, reinforce the match between the job and your skills and interests, and any job adaptations the job requires, to help guide your reference in the event they are asked to verify your qualifications and your ability to handle the job.

As we mentioned before, using references is tricky if they are not absolutely convinced that your blindness would not affect your job performance. If you're not certain how they would respond to questions about your blindness, briefly describe how you plan to handle the job, and ask for any questions they may have about your disability.

JOB-HUNTING ERRORS

Before we leave the subject of job-search tactics, study these "Ten Major Mistakes" that job seekers make which were compiled from several surveys of prominent recruiters and were summarized in Jack Erdlen's book CAREERSEARCH.

1. *Poor Resume*

This document is used as a screening device by most employers. If poorly prepared, it can quickly eliminate you from consideration. The resume should describe education and experience in a concise, well-written format. Accomplishments should be emphasized over duties and responsibilities.

2. *Failure to Network*

Friends, acquaintances, and their referrals are the most effective job sources for most candidates, especially in senior-level positions. They are often overlooked or avoided for a variety of unacceptable reasons. Job hunters must be aggressive in developing and pursuing leads from these contacts.

3. *Limiting Job Sources*

Classified ads, employment agencies, executive search firms, and college placement offices are valuable sources. Any dislikes or prejudices should be disregarded in favor of using them to complete a total job search. Thousands of candidates are hired annually through these sources.

4. *"Canned" Approach*

Pre-printed cover letters, stereotypical telephone calls, and generic resumes are viewed negatively by most employers who feel "If the candidate takes shortcuts in creating an initial impression, what can be expected after he (she) becomes an employee?"

5. *A 12-15 Hour Work Week*

For the unemployed, a job search should be a continual 40-hour per week proposition. For the employed, new priorities must include the commitment of personal and vacation time to this effort. Candidates often "run out of steam" after a short period, and a 12-15 hour search week will not normally produce desirable results.

6. *Inadequate Interview Preparation*

Each situation must be viewed as a separate challenge. A presentation that is impressive to one firm can easily fall short for another. No two interviews or corporations are alike.

Responses must be timely and flexible and must address the specific needs of the employer, and this approach requires preparation.

7. *Poor Interviewing Techniques*

An honest "give and take" relationship must be established during the interview. Candidates are encouraged to exchange information while listening attentively, selling themselves, and demonstrating enthusiasm for the job and the company.

8. *Restricted Job Search*

A "worst case" approach should be implemented, if possible. Restriction on geographic locations, commuting times, size and type of company, and other personal preferences should be secondary to examining all of the available opportunities. An offer can always be declined if it is judged to be unattractive, or if a better situation develops. Financial and professional pressures can also change your outlook at a later date and make the offer more feasible.

9. *Negative Attitude*

Candidates who "have all the answers," who criticize their managers and "second guess" their employers, are seldom invited for second interviews. Previous performance and a negative attitude are seen as predictors of future performance.

10. *Poor Physical Appearance*

While candidates are hardly expected to be look-alikes for TV and movie stars, there is no excuse for poor grooming. If an individual does not demonstrate self-respect by creating a positive image, he (she) is judged to be incompatible.

COMPLETING AN APPLICATION FORM

Few things are more discouraging than having your carefully crafted resume brushed aside by a personnel manager who asks, instead, that you complete a standard employment application form. How can this be?

Just when you get a grip on what makes you so interesting, what makes you unique, someone forces you to squeeze your rich life history into a standardized, boring, nondescript mold.

And so it goes.

Nevertheless, employment application forms are standard operating equipment, so you should know how to handle them. Here are a few tips:

¤ *Ask for assistance.* Under the "reasonable accommodation" requirements which are included in most EEO and Affirmative Action laws and regulations, you can reasonably ask one of the secretaries in the employment office to help you fill out the application. The only problem with this approach is that you do not know if that particular secretary is neat and accurate. You might try the next approach.

¤ *Ask if you can take the application form home.* If you want to be certain that your application conveys the excellent impression you want to make, you can ask to take the application home. Plus, it gives you more time to think. If you do, make a couple of photocopies of the form to practice on before filling in the original form.

¤ *Use the well-crafted language of your resume.* If the sentences and phrases in your resume are as concise and action-oriented as they should be, transfer them to your application form.

¤ *Don't lie on the application form*. If, after you are hired, your employer discovers that you lied on the application, you could be fired. If you have unexplained gaps in your employment history, mention them in a positive way; for example, if you have a period of rehabilitation in your record, say something like "Took a leave of absence for one year in order to acquire some job-related skills." You can elaborate on that statement during the interview.

¤ *Do not leave any questions unanswered*. If the employer asks for a salary history, it's best to say that your salary is "open to negotiation," rather than showing your salary needs so early in the game.

¤ *Think before you answer*. The wrong answer to a question like "Why did you leave your last job?" can raise serious doubts in the mind of the employer. Here's what Jack Erdlen says about the responses some job applicants give to this question, and the doubts they raise among employers:

Lack of work: Was this really the case, or was the individual simply not able to do it?

Layoff: Was the applicant the only person laid off, or was it a major layoff?

Better job: Will this person be leaving soon for another, better job?

Personal reasons: Drugs or drinking problems? Nervous breakdown?

No room for advancement: Is this view objective, or is the applicant not promotable?

Poor health: High absentee factor? High medical claims?

Personality conflicts with supervisor: Are these conflicts an ongoing problem?

More money: Will the applicant continually press for salary increases? Does the applicant have an inflated opinion of his/her real worth?

Uninteresting, routine work: Does this person become bored easily? Is keeping this applicant happy a full-time job?

The point is, you want to answer the question honestly, but you want to allay any doubts about yourself in an interviewer's mind. According to Joyce Lain Kennedy, you should simply write "Opportunity," implying that you moved on for bigger and better things.

As you already know, equal employment opportunity and affirmative action regulations prohibit employers from asking questions that are not strictly job-related. For example, employers used to ask on the application form "Do you have any physical or mental disability?"

That question has been replaced with "Is there anything that you think would impede you from doing the job?" If the answer is no, say no. You don't have to mention your blindness anywhere on the application, unless you choose to do so.

¤ *Have names, addresses, and phone numbers of work references handy*. Most applications ask for specific work references. You will also need the specific dates of your various jobs and educational accomplishments.

Don't underestimate the importance of the employment application, even if it appears to be a sterile presentation of you and your accomplishments. Every step in the job-search process counts, for or against you.

LONG-DISTANCE JOB HUNTING

The more willing you are to relocate, the better your chances are of finding the right job for you. Unfortunately, because of society's misconceptions about blindness, many employers will presume that blindness and job-related mobility are incompatible. This reluctance to view blind people as dynamic and mobile is, perhaps, exemplified most strikingly by the United States Department of State, which still excludes qualified blind (and other severely disabled) individuals from employment in the Foreign Service.

Still, the trend toward greater labor market mobility is a fact. You'd better get used to the idea of not only packing up and moving *for* a job, but packing up and moving *on* the job. Here are some strategies for conducting a long-distance job search:

1. *Plan to Travel to Your Destination.*

At some point, you will need to visit the area of your choice for job interviews, informational interviews, visits to employment agencies, research sessions at local libraries, and get-togethers with networking contacts. Plan to stay at least a week, preferably longer.

2. *Your Written Communication Must Be First-Rate.*

To keep your phone expenses down, you will be forced to rely on your written communication. It must be very, very good. The fact is, unless you have some unique and highly-sought-after skill, or unless you can pull in $45,000 plus in salary, chances are good that employers won't want to incur the expenses associated with an out-of-town (or -state) applicant. We mentioned earlier that employers like to minimize risks; naturally, bringing someone on board from a distance appears more risky than hiring an outside candidate locally.

One way to keep the travel costs down is to target companies that are headquartered in your destination city, but which have a branch office in the city where you live. That way, if the local manager is sufficiently impressed, he or she may convince headquarters to fly you out at the company's expense.

3. *Target and Focus Your Research.*

Taking on a new city is, as kids would say, an "awesome" task. The only way you can manage what seems like an overwhelming task is to target and focus your job research. Here are a few ways to do that:

¤ Subscribe to the local papers of your targeted city. If it's a major city, check a nearby newsstand or school or public library. Otherwise, call the city and subscribe through the mail. Remember, too, that national newspapers, such as *The Wall Street Journal*, often publish regional editions, rather than a single national one. And don't forget about magazines that focus on particular cities or states, such as *Texas Monthly*, *The Washingtonian*, and *Manhattan Inc.*, as well as the more specialized ones, such as *Indianapolis Business Journal* and *New York Woman*.

¤ Purchase the Yellow Pages directory of your destination city from your local telephone company. It's loaded with information about employers in the area.

¤ Contact employment agencies and executive search firms, found in the membership directory of the National Association of Personnel Consultants and in the many directories of executive recruiters that are available, like the *Directory of Executive Recruiters*.

¤ Study "Job Bank" books, which list and describe major employers in the area. Bob Adams, Inc., and Contacts Influential are two such publishers.

¤ Is there a toll-free employment hotline which lists current openings in local government or academe? Check with the civil service department, or any of the universities in your destination city.

¤ Contact the local chamber of commerce and the public library in your targeted area, to inquire about the overall economic situation in that city and the nature and scope of their job-related information.

¤ Network through the professional society or trade association to which you belong; obtain listings of members who live and work in your desired location.

¤ Similarly, contact the alumni office of your alma mater.

¤ Other good resources are national organizations of the blind, which have local chapters in most regions across the country. The Job Opportunities for the Blind (JOB) Program is a good place to check.

¤ Don't forget friends, relatives, and acquaintances who may live in your targeted area.

4. *Relocation Is A Family Affair.*

If you have a family, involve them in the process. Your spouse may be quite content job-wise, and your children will probably not want to leave their friends and the school they know. To complicate matters, there's the stress of house-selling and -finding, locating suitable schools, and so forth. Some employers offer help with relocation expenses; be sure you know exactly what kind of help before you pack up and leave the nest. And don't forget about realty companies and full-service relocation consultants who are trained to help with relocation headaches.

SO WHAT ARE YOU WAITING FOR?

Well, there you have it. No doubt, the job search process is a great deal more complicated than you thought. The more approaches you use, the better your chances are of finding the right job for you.

You now know 14 ways to tap into the open job market, and the four essential steps for uncovering the hidden job market.

In order to stay afloat and headed in the right direction, you need to keep pace with a constantly changing job market. The better informed you are about the working world around you, the more it will seem that pure "luck" is following you around. ¤

Chapter 5
What Do Employers Think?

What do employers think about hiring a blind person?

Plenty.

And they're nervous . . . very nervous.

Too little public education has been done to reverse the DISabled image of blindness that most employers carry around in their heads. As a blind job seeker, you need to know what bothers employers most about hiring a blind person, in order to prepare a strategy for breaking through the resistance and winning the job.

Knowledge is power. It's better to know what the person sitting on the other side of the desk may be thinking—ahead of time. The legendary American general George S. Patton, as depicted in the movie bearing his name, after winning a decisive military victory against German field marshal Rommel during World War II, shook his fist in the air in triumph and shouted, "*Rommel, you bastard, I read your book!*" He knew something about strategy.

Because most employers would be reluctant to share their deepest concerns with you, for fear of a potential law suit, we granted several employers anonymity and asked them, for the purpose of this book, to be very honest. They were. Sometimes painfully so. Even though we interviewed the "best" of the bunch—employers who were able to see beyond their prejudices and who *have* hired qualified blind people—their comments still carry some of the same assumptions about blindness that have plagued blind job seekers for generations.

For instance, one employer remarked that he would not take a blind person on a tour of the company if the staff had not been "warned" of the applicant's blindness. This employer probably wouldn't dream of making a similar comment about a black person, or a woman. Two decades ago, he might have.

It's important to remember that the interests of the employer and the interests of the blind job seeker may be at odds. Women in the labor market understand this very well. They understand that most employers have concerns about child care and maternity leave and may try to coax this information out of a woman during an interview. Women have a choice: They may choose to not address this issue, feeling that child care is their business, or they may choose to share this information because that approach best serves their interests.

You have choices, too.

There is a danger in presenting such a limited number of interviews with employers. This small sampling may not be representative of the whole—but, in a general sense, we think it is.

Here is what a few employers said, verbatim.

§

Interview with a Personnel Manager for a Large High-Tech Company

Have you ever interviewed and hired a blind job applicant?

Yes, both.

How would a disabled job applicant gain entry into the company?

It's the same for all applicants. We don't have special people working with disabled applicants, if that's what you mean. No matter who you are, you would find that it's a long process—usually five to seven interviews.

230

What advice would you give to a blind job applicant trying to get into your company?

First, I would say you must have the necessary skills. If you're not sure what those are, FIND OUT BEFORE YOU COME IN. You must have some work experience—do volunteer work, internships, summer jobs, anything, but don't come in and say that you've never worked. We are a tough company to get into, no matter who you are.

Don't come in here saying you want a job with computers and then say you don't like technical things in the next breath, like one blind job applicant did. You must know what your transferable skills are BEFORE you come in for the interview. Otherwise, don't waste my time.

How would you feel if a blind job applicant appeared for a scheduled interview and you did not know beforehand that the applicant was blind?

I would avoid surprises. You would *not* be getting off to a good start. The average supervisor would be set back and would need some time to regain composure. They would probably be uncomfortable showing the applicant around, which typically is done. Usually, you take the applicant around and introduce him or her to the other managers; you might not do that in this situation because you hadn't properly prepared the other managers.

People don't like surprises.

What concerns supervisors most about hiring a blind applicant?

A supervisor's biggest fear is the unknown, not that the person can't do the job. They have the qualifications to do the job, or they would not have been called in for an interview. The supervisor is thinking, "What am I going to do? Will I have to spend more time with this person? Will the other employees resent it if I do? How will the other co-workers feel about this hire?"

The blind job applicant *must* take the initiative in bringing up issues of job accommodation. If you have your own equipment, mention it—anything to reduce the barriers to employment. Employers prefer an "easy" qualified hire to a "difficult" one. For example, if two equally qualified candidates applied for a job, and one lived nearby and the other one would have to relocate (with the employer paying relocation costs), we would hire the closer one.

Money for job accommodation comes out of the individual line manager's budget, which penalizes the manager for hiring a disabled employee. We have been trying to get that policy changed by having one general company fund to draw from, but it hasn't happened. It's just one more barrier to getting a disabled person on board.

What different avenues exist for getting one's foot in the door?

I would pursue both personnel and line managers. If you talk with a recruiter, it could just be exploratory; in other words, maybe there isn't a particular job opening at that time, but you could use that opportunity to find out more about the company.

Whatever you do, take the initiative. Rehab isn't the way to go. You can't just let them do all the work . . . that wouldn't impress me. You must do it yourself.

Are employers concerned about mobility issues?

Yes, but if you got to the interview by yourself, you would probably address that concern. Time is short in an interview. You must cover your skills and describe how you are going to do the job.

We will be proposing a strategy in the book, and would like your comments on it. The strategy is this: Because the typical manager cannot envision a blind person doing most jobs, we are suggesting to blind applicants that they identify three blind individuals in the country (or in their area) who are doing the same type of job. Then, we are telling them to ask these three individuals to ask their immediate supervisors if they would mind being contacted by prospective employers about how their blind subordinates handle their jobs. What do you think?

I think that would be very helpful; it's a selling point. But you must be very certain that these three individuals' supervisors really do think they are doing the job. I think if you could find three supervisors who wholeheartedly endorsed their blind employees, it could reduce the prospective employer's concerns.

Interview with the Personnel Manager of a Large International Manufacturing Firm, Who Is Himself Disabled

Have you ever interviewed and hired a blind job applicant?

We started hiring people with disabilities back in the Fifties. It's part of our corporate philosophy. We think of ourselves as very progressive in this area; we are among the best. We have plenty of financial resources for both people and programs.

Of course, hiring people with disabilities may be "old hat" to some of us, but it's still new to new supervisors. People have to be educated about this on an ongoing basis, and sometimes that gets tiring . . . .

How successful are your visually impaired employees?

It's a mixed bag, of course. We've had people who have not worked out, and then we have a deaf-blind person who puts out 120%. And we have another person who required enormous amounts of training, but who is working out nicely.

What employment problems have you had with these employees?

I'll be honest. It takes a lot of resources, both financially and time-wise, to make this work. In the beginning, we, too, had stereotypic jobs that blind people could do, like darkroom stuff. When we started looking at other jobs that visually impaired employees could do, some of them required investments in equipment which cost quite a bit of money. We brought in consultants and relied heavily on the local support groups, like Project with Industry. Training is another area that takes money and time. But we were committed to doing this, and it worked.

Did you like having local resources, like Project with Industry, available for consultation?

Yes, it gives you a sense of comfortableness. They come in and say, "Sure, yes, this can be done. A blind person can do that."

How would you feel about a job applicant who appeared at your door for a scheduled interview, and who was blind and had not mentioned it beforehand?

I'd be a little pissed off. I wouldn't recommend surprising anyone.

But could it work for some people?

Well, let me think about that.

IF you had the necessary skills and training; IF you were comfortable with your disability and with people; IF you could demonstrate, in detail, how you would handle the job; IF you knew exactly what you wanted and had the requisite experience, MAYBE you could get away with it.

For example, if you came here and wanted a job in customer service, well, we already have a blind person working in that capacity, so people wouldn't be too surprised. But if it were in some new area and the job applicant didn't know how he/she was going to do the job, I probably would not be able to continue the interview. I'd have to reschedule it after I had had some time to think.

The other problem with not disclosing is the fact that I like to take prospective applicants around the building to meet others. If they have a disability, I prepare the other employees in advance. If I hadn't done that, I probably would not take the person around. That's a real minus in a job interview situation.

What are the employer's concerns about hiring a blind person?

The greatest barrier is, of course, attitudinal. Can this lady get to the ladies' room? We're past that in this company. We know that many people have a disability. We have people who drink too much, women whose husbands beat them, people who chronically arrive late, people who don't get along with others . . . these are all disabilities.

The problem is, most employers think that about 10% of all jobs could be done by a blind person. Blind people probably think it's 80%. The truth is somewhere in between. That's a big gap in perception.

What do you think of the assistance which rehabilitation agencies provide to blind job applicants?

We're all counseling each other to death. I'm particularly tired of people with disabilities going into counseling jobs to counsel other people with disabilities. It's such a closed circle.

Support agencies are good for helping *employers* identify and accommodate work sites; I'm not sure they're so good for the applicants.

What advice would you like to give to blind job seekers?

I would tell blind job seekers three things:
1. Sighted people are a mixed bag, too, just like you. Some are wonderful, some are horrible. Some are afraid and just don't know how to handle the situation, others do. You need a lot of patience. And the job never ends . . . the job of educating them.
2. Sighted people are going to screw up (treat you badly). It's your cross to bear. Do the best you can and get on with life.
3. There isn't much time to dwell on your anger. It's legitimate, even justified, but don't let it consume you. Who wants to hire an angry, nasty person? Would you?

Interview with the Chief Executive Officer of a Bank

Have you ever interviewed and hired a blind job applicant?

Yes, twice.

How did that happen?

Well, we had been talking for some time about getting someone in to handle telephone calls about mortgage rates and other bank matters. Hank, the president at the time, said he knew this blind woman who had a "terrific brain," and asked me if I would try her in the position. I said, "Let's give it a try."

Sounds like a pretty easy decision, especially since you had never hired a blind person before.

It's really the attitude of the bank. We have never been a staid type of organization; we're not right down the line here. There is no such thing as "the way things are done around here." There's a high degree of individualism here; sometimes you might call it zoo-like.

Did you prepare the other employees for the addition of a blind co-worker?

No, no fanfare. She just showed up.

Were people uncomfortable?

Yes, but nothing terrible ever happened. Just subtle things, like people not knowing what to do, offering too much help and unnecessary help. You know, they had their own preconceived notions about blind people.

Do you wish you had gathered the troops together to discuss the new worker before she arrived?

I think you should wait and see what happens. What happened here was that one person, who seemed to be the most comfortable, sort of showed her around the first few days.

What channels would you suggest a blind applicant use to get into your bank?

Well, in this case, it was a personal referral, which is the strongest channel for anyone but especially for someone who is blind, I would think. It depends on the organization and the people. For example, if she had contacted a branch manager for a position here, the manager probably wouldn't know anything about what a blind person could do at the bank. The people in Personnel would know much more about the different types of jobs at the bank. Managers can't always visualize all of the kinds of jobs we have here, like Personnel can. But personnel people are extremely busy and can't exert a lot of special effort on someone's behalf.

The best way is through a personal referral, but I wouldn't rule out Personnel if you can clearly define your skills. If a person who were blind came in and said, "Here's what I can do for you, is this something you need?", it would probably work out.

You knew before the interview that this woman was blind. What if she came in for the interview and you didn't know?

I'd be a little burned. You want people to be straight with you. The assumption is always that the employer has it made and the applicant has it tough. Well, maybe the employer hasn't had such a great day, or year, either. They deserve some respect, too.

So this person appears at the door and all of a sudden you've got another minicrisis on your hands. "Will this person sue me if I don't treat him/her right? How much longer will it take to discuss the disability-related questions? Can I? How much more work is it going to take to find a job here for this person? Who's going to do that work?" And so on. You're thinking, "I'm working too hard to be treated like this."

It's a matter of trust. Trust is very important these days. In fact, one of the first questions you ask yourself is, can I trust this prospective employee?

What if the person did not mention being blind on the resume, but, after being contacted for an interview, did bring it up?

That would be fair. That would be okay.

What if the person mentioned on the resume or over the phone that they had a disability, but didn't specify blindness?

Disabled means, to most people, that you don't walk too well so you can't handle the stairs. Or you have a heart condition and can barely show up for work. It doesn't have a positive connotation.

What should the blind job applicant say about his/her blindness during the interview?

If somebody walks into this company, with or without experience, and they're blind, *blindness is the biggest part of the interview.*

Two things need to be covered:
   1. This is what I can do for you . . . .
   2. This is the kind of person I am . . . .

One of the biggest complaints of employers today is that employees don't give a damn. If you come in saying you want to work, and you have a good strong work ethic and a good attitude, you stand out. Sell yourself as having these qualities:
   I will give a little more effort than someone else . . . .
   I'm going to work very hard for you . . . .
   I want to be successful . . . .

What if a blind job applicant brought someone along with them to the interview?

The kiss of death. And bringing a spouse is worse than bringing a mother.

What about someone in your company escorting a prospective job applicant to your office for the interview?

Sometimes a big deal is made of this . . . with the security officer getting involved, like it's a security risk. That's unfortunate.

I think a blind person should not hesitate to ask for regular, sensible assistance. Anybody would expect that a blind interviewee would not be able to find a strange office without some assistance. Actually, it's the same for *all* applicants; usually my secretary goes out and gets them. This is better than refusing assistance and wandering around the building, lost, with everyone becoming more and more uncomfortable. It is assumed by any intelligent person that some things will be different. Don't sweat the small stuff.

Is work experience important?

We don't care if you have a Master's degree; if you don't have any work experience, we don't want you.

What if a blind job applicant came in with a job idea and offered to work as a volunteer for three months?

I would be impressed. I'd give it a shot. I like that approach—it's a "let me prove it to you" approach.

What about job accommodation?

That's difficult, and we certainly have had problems with that. I think the employee or the State Rehabilitation Agency should assume responsibility for any hardware or major piece of equipment; say, anything over $1,000. The company could pick up the rest, like software.

If they're a big company, maybe they could do more. It depends on their size and resources. Generally, I think it should be limited to a few hundred dollars. The result is that the employer feels better about the placement.

What if a blind job applicant gave you the names of two other blind individuals doing the same job elsewhere, and the names of their supervisors for you to call. Would that be helpful?

Yes. That would be effective. I mean, let's face it, the employer realizes that this is an unusual situation that requires some unusual techniques.

What would help convince you to hire a blind applicant?

The person must be able to describe, very concretely, how he or she would do the job. If the person has a piece of the necessary technology, so much the better. I remember being very impressed with the equipment one applicant brought in with her.

Second, I would say, be realistic. I'm not going to try out for the Red Sox tomorrow, no matter how much I want it. The applicant should know what he or she really can do. The reason the woman who worked here was so successful—she has since been recruited to work at another company, with a promotion—was that she lived in the real world. She knew what she could do, she knew what she could do in a different way, and she knew what she couldn't do.

Third, know something about the company. It doesn't even need to be that much. People come in here to apply for a job because they bank here and "like the atmosphere." They know something about the company.

Last, if the person convinces me that he or she is going to give me a real effort, I like that.

What advice would you give to blind job applicants?

Recognize that you have a handicap; it's real. Don't sweep it under the rug. Yes, some people will think it's worse than it is, and you can explain that.

Interview with a Personnel Manager for an Insurance Company

Have you ever interviewed and hired a blind job applicant?

I have, yes.

Did a blind applicant just walk through the door, or did you recruit them?

Our CEO sits on the board of an agency for the blind. He agreed to hire a blind person, and had already identified the candidate.

Had you hired people with disabilities before?

Yes, we had hired several people who were deaf.

How has the blind employee worked out?

Very well. John is a pretty loose, outgoing kind of guy. He makes people around him comfortable, so he set the tone. It wasn't difficult at all.

Were other employees concerned?

Yes, there were concerns. Not in the telemarketing department, where he was going to work—they're a young, crazy, outgoing bunch of people—but elsewhere in the company, people were nervous. There were some concerns that he would be treated differently.

How did you handle this?

We contacted the local rehabilitation agency, and they showed us a film that told us how to behave—it's a film where everyone is overly helpful, and everyone started laughing. Later, after John had been here for a while, people asked to see the film again. We did some educating.

Was this approach helpful?

Very. Not knowing things, like how to walk with John to the lunchroom, not knowing when he wants help and when he doesn't, not knowing how to identify ourselves, all these things were brought out in the film. We could laugh about it and about ourselves.

You know, people were just uncomfortable not knowing what to do. You don't like to feel uncomfortable. Even after the film, John had to continue to educate people. People were petting his dog and the dog wasn't responding to his commands; he walked into a couple of walls . . . . John finally had to speak up about a few of these things.

What concerns did you have about hiring a blind person?

My first concern was getting through the interview—I was very uncomfortable. Once we got started, John put me at ease and my apprehension just left.

As far as his working here, one concern was how the other employees would relate to him. But John settled that quickly enough; he's one of the team.

We were also concerned about how he was going to do the job, but again John settled that question. He was very knowledgeable about the job and he didn't really need a lot of equipment—just a tape recorder and his memory. We did put everything on tape for him; he said he used to fall asleep at home listening to our voices. His memory is incredible; he knows the dental plan rates by heart, by territory—I don't know that. He remembers everything.

John's biggest concern was, how do you read rates over the phone? Generally, the job doesn't require that, but if he gets stuck, he has to turn the call over to someone else.

What would you consider a reasonable expense for a job accommodation?

I don't know, but not over $3,000. When you get over that figure, you start to wonder if it's really worth it.

Imagine, if you can, that John arrived for the interview and you had not been told beforehand that he was blind.

Well, of course I'd be surprised. I guess a little off guard. From a personal standpoint, I'd be thinking, "Why didn't you tell me?" I couldn't ask him that question, either.

So, the interview would probably be very awkward. My concern would be, why didn't he tell me and does this mean he's going to be extremely defensive if I say anything about his blindness? If I say something wrong, will he wallop me?

In other words, I would see this as an "attitude" problem. If he came in like this, what is his expectation as an employee? Am I just expected to automatically accommodate him in any way he wants?

I would probably waste at least half the interview just adjusting to the situation, and miss out on the real point of the interview.

The other thing is, by the time we've screened the applications, selected a few possibilities, talked with the applicant over the phone, and scheduled the interview, we've already told the line supervisor he's coming. Well, now you've got to inform the supervisor that—surprise—the applicant is blind. Of course, that doesn't make you look good; the supervisor is thinking, "Why didn't you tell me?" It's a reflection on me as a member of Personnel. It means I didn't screen the applicant properly, which is my job. But what could I have done, asked the applicant over the phone, "Are you blind?"

A dozen questions would be running through my mind. How is he ever going to learn everything? How could he do the job? But there's no time to prepare for that; the applicant is already in your office. People are afraid of law suits, so you have to be careful. There would be no time to check out these legalities, in terms of what you can ask a job applicant relevant to his disability.

What if an applicant did not mention blindness on his resume, but did tell you after the interview had been scheduled but before you actually met?

That would be okay. If any employer cancelled the interview after that, they could justifiably be sued for discrimination.

What unexpected issues came up?

We never thought about John's dog. It turns out there's an individual who has allergies . . . and it has been a BIG issue. First, the question was, where is *she* going to sit? We put John at one end of the room, and her at the other. We also put a vent over her head. But then she was unhappy because she didn't want to be away from everyone; it's a team environment. And she couldn't get to the ladies' room without going past the dog.

Then there was the problem with the coffee lady. She goes around at breaks and brings coffee and donuts for sale. She would break down around John and say, "Oh, I'll pay for it dear (how can he afford it?)," when John was making more money than she was.

Another problem was transportation. There isn't any public transportation around here. So we made arrangements for the company mail truck to pick John up and take him home at night. It works fine. We're a young company and most of the people are under 30, so you don't want to be committed to giving someone a ride home each night. You may want to go out after work, and don't want to feel that you left a blind person stranded.

What advice would you give to blind job seekers?

Know what you want and what you can do. Tell me what you need, because only you know.

Interview with the Director of a Data-Processing Department for a Large Health-Care Company

Have you ever interviewed or hired a blind job applicant?

I've interviewed a half-dozen, and hired one.

How did this happen?

It was something I wanted to do. My mother is disabled, and I wanted to hire a blind person in my department. I don't know why I decided the person's disability should be blindness—maybe because I think it is so difficult.

I made the decision and started to do a little research. I heard that there was a blind woman working as a programmer for an electric company in Ohio. (I didn't know there were blind computer programmers right in town.) I flew down there to interview her and her supervisor. Well, I walked into a hornet's nest. The blind employee was unhappy, and her superiors were unhappy with her, but they weren't talking to each other. They *did* talk to me! I became an intermediary. I spent the whole day there and taped the interviews. She thought she was doing a fine job; they thought she was doing, essentially, nothing.

I realized, from talking to these people, that there were problems I had not considered, like transportation, guide dogs—I'm not crazy about dogs—equipment, and so on. Apparently, the woman in Ohio fell asleep during the day. Her supervisors thought this was because she was blind; you know, like sitting in the dark all day makes you sleepy. I didn't know if that were true or not.

Well, before I moved much further on this "quest," I was promoted and transferred to a new department. That was good, and bad. Good, because my new boss sat on the board of a local rehabilitation agency, and bad, because this was a new department and I knew I couldn't rock the boat until I had established myself.

Once I had, I alerted Personnel that I was interested in interviewing blind applicants for a programming position.

Several applicants were sent from the state rehabilitation agency; I interviewed seven candidates. Normally, there is an entrance examination given to programmers (by Personnel), but this was waived temporarily.

Personnel had already done some prescreening, and then my boss and I interviewed several candidates. It was tough. I wrestled with myself: Was I rejecting any of these candidates because they weren't qualified, or because they were blind? None of them was right. It's a team environment around here, so interpersonal skills are a must.

What didn't seem right about these candidates?

They had chips on their shoulders.

What exactly does that mean? Can you describe it?

They felt the world owed them a living because they were blind. They were very pushy, they just kept saying, "I know I can do the job." They thought they could do it, so what I thought seemed irrelevant. Just because they had the desire, I was supposed to give them a job. Just because they had written one simple program for the PC, they felt qualified to do the job. I would ask them, "What do you think you'll be doing every day?" They would say, "I'll be programming." I'd respond, "90% of the time you won't be writing programs." They didn't have a clue about the job; they really didn't know what they were talking about.

What impressed you about the person you hired?

I knew in five minutes that I wanted Bill. His presence, his appearance, his willingness to speak to the issues—*he was comfortable with himself.* He understood what he *couldn't* do, too. I asked him, for example, what had been the most difficult part of his computer-programming course, and he said, "The reading requirements. I had to wait for my reader." But he added, "The compensating skill that I have is a good memory. I can remember the requirements without looking them up again."

How did the company react to Bill's coming on board?

The environment here is very conservative, very traditional. There was no receptiveness to this at all. I met with some team managers and explained that I had interviewed Bill and that he would be available. At first, no one responded. Then, one day, one of the female managers came into my office and wanted to know more about Bill. We spent two hours talking about him. If Carol had not come forward, I don't think anyone else would have.

Carol went back to her team and talked with them. They had a lot of questions. How does he do this, or that? What if we use the word "see," etc.? I was as ignorant about this as anyone. In the end, Carol agreed to interview him with me.

How did the interview go?

The people in Personnel gave him the wrong directions . . . they sent him through the wrong street entrance, and he ended up on the loading dock. But he still got to my office on time, and without going through security! We were very impressed.

Carol wasn't just uncomfortable asking questions, she was uncomfortable, period. In fact, she was a nervous wreck. Still, she agreed to the hire.

Do you think you could have asked the other managers to just meet this guy once before making a decision?

In my old department, yes. They would have done it for me. But this department was a different environment; you have to analyze the management culture. The culture can differ even within the same department, depending on the players.

The least sympathetic were the men . . . the women were better. They seemed more willing to give it a try.

What about job accommodation once the decision was made?

That was a big problem. First, the IBM equipment that we ordered for Bill was going to take nine months to arrive. I couldn't hire him until we had the equipment. Bill didn't know whether to wait or to start looking somewhere else. The interview was in October, and Bill didn't come on board until March. It would have been July, but we found another blind employee working in another department (I didn't even know that) who loaned him a piece of equipment until his arrived.

What about the expense of the equipment?

It cost about $3,500, which wasn't a problem for us. We are used to buying equipment, and our purchases are state-of-the-art.

Did you prepare the staff in any way for Bill's arrival?

Yes. We had someone from the state rehabilitation agency come in and talk to the staff before Bill came. The staff needed to know that there was support available. They could have listened to me, but I didn't know anything, either.

These are data-processing people—very inquisitive people. I mean, they had a list of 20 questions.

Do you think you could have handled this some other way, like asking Bill to talk to people about these things?

No, I don't think people would have been comfortable asking Bill these questions. They would now, but not then. It was very helpful to have an outside person come in. Now, of course, I could do this myself.

So, do you think the rehabilitation agency serves a good purpose in the job-search process?

I was asked last summer to sit on an employer panel for a seminar sponsored by the state rehabilitation agency. I told the counselors their job should be to *educate employers*. I told them they should *not* be a support person for the job applicant, but a third party for the employer. If the applicant can't get through the process by him- or herself, then forget it. I told them the clients they had sent me came through with chips on their shoulders, and that they should have talked to their clients about their attitudes. I told them they sent clients who weren't qualified, and that if they were in the employment business, they would be *out* of business. I wasn't too popular that day.

What do you think about a job applicant's showing up at your office without telling you ahead of time that he/she is blind?

That's easy. They wouldn't get the job. That's the same question the rehabilitation counselors asked me that day. And they argued with me. I told them, "You folks don't live in the real world. We're human. We all have our own inhibitions and hang-ups, and you can't ignore that. You'll never know, if you try that tactic, whether you didn't get the job because the interviewer was in a state of shock, or because you didn't have the skills. If the interviewer doesn't know ahead of time that the job applicant is blind, you can forget it. I don't believe the person will get the job. I'll guarantee it."

I need to be prepared. I pride myself on being prepared. That's how I got here. It's a whole different set of questions and issues, and I need to prepare for it. I prepare for all of my interviews. I would be so shocked, if a blind person came in unannounced, that I would spend the entire interview just trying to recover. That's just not going to work.

You don't hire people just because they have the skills. You also hire them because you like them. And you're not going to like them very much if you're upset. Everyone has the "Oh, my God" kind of feeling the first time they meet a blind person. It may not be right, but it's the natural reaction. We're human, too.

What if the person did not disclose on the resume, but notified the interviewer by phone before the interview?

That would be okay. As long as I know ahead of the interview.

Do you believe, based on your experience, that a blind employee can compete on equal terms?

If a person is just an average worker, no. It's going to take longer to do some tasks. The question is, what compensating skills does the blind employee have that can balance the scale? If the person is slower, but more accurate, that tips the scale. If the person has better interpersonal skills, that makes a difference.

What final advice would you like to give?

I want to hear how self-sufficient you are. I'm willing to go the extra yard, but I want to hear that you are, too. The woman in Ohio has a special appraisal form; she gets special treatment. I don't want that.

Interview with the Personnel Director of a Large International Computer-Products Firm

Have you ever interviewed and hired a blind job applicant?

Yes, several.

Was your company receptive?

Quite frankly, we had a mandate to hire six disabled people by the end of the year; we get government contracts. We had relatively no experience in this area. We contacted the local Project with Industry (PWI) and worked with them. They came in and did site surveys in all the departments and identified several jobs that could be done by blind people.

How have these employees worked out?

We hired three blind people, two entry-level positions and one advanced. Two have worked out very well, and one is a problem. The fellow who isn't working out brought his mother to the interview; we should have seen that as a sign.

How easy or difficult was the process?

It was difficult. I think it would be very difficult for a company that had never hired a blind person to do it without some help, like we had from PWI. We just didn't feel secure about the situation. We liked having access to people who did feel secure about all this. I think it's critical to have a support system for *employers*. It's too difficult to go it alone . . . there are too many questions, and personnel people are paranoid about discrimination suits if they ask too many questions of the job applicant.

Did you use the local rehab agency?

Rehab people know nothing. Our experience with vocational rehabilitation people is dismal. They send clients who are not job-ready, and you have to deal with too many agencies.

The people at Project with Industry sent a woman to talk to our managers and to answer some of their questions. We didn't know she was visually impaired, too. One of the managers asked, "How will a blind person follow my training sessions when I use a blackboard?", and then the manager got up and gave a demonstration. So the woman from PWI said, "Look, I can't see the blackboard and I followed everything you just did. I went through four years of college and could never see the blackboard." That sold him. That's the kind of extra support we needed. There were a lot of issues like that that we felt we needed to iron out. Now we know, but back then we didn't.

What would be the best approach for entry into this company?

It's very difficult to get an approval to hire. We're controlled by head count. We're allowed to have 3,497 people on board, and not one over that. In this case, because the company needed to hire disabled people, we were given permission to increase a manager's head count by one if they hired a disabled person.

Let's face it—that was the motivation. People avoid risks. Managers avoid risks. Companies avoid risks. Hiring a blind person implies risk.

How can a blind job applicant work around this resistance?

Networking. In fact, the reason networking works so well is that IT REDUCES RISK. For example, if someone calls me, someone whom I trust, and says they know somebody who could do such and such . . . I trust that person, so I'm likely to give this applicant the benefit of the doubt. It's not favoritism, it's a chance to reduce the risk factor. Someone called me this morning . . . they have an intern who's good, and she wants me to keep my eyes open for something. I will.

The other important element is work experience. I look at my own daughter's situation. Several summers ago, she started working at Burger King. My husband and I thought, Big deal. But we saw that she was really learning some skills, such as selling: "Do you want fries with that?" That's important. And she got performance appraisals, something she hadn't known about. She saw what was important to employers. Then she moved to waitressing. My husband and I marveled at the way she treated customers—she was always so shy at home. During college, she got a summer internship where she interviewed politicians and important sports figures. She learned a tremendous amount about the networks. Now she's working as a volunteer with a TV station.

When she goes out looking for her first full-time permanent job after college, she will be bringing an enormous amount of experience and some polished skills. I realize now that this type of work education is absolutely essential to any job seeker.

What impressed you about the blind applicants you hired?

We were impressed with the candidate who had graduated from a regular computer-programming course. We also hired someone who had attended a special program for the blind, and he hasn't worked out. Now we realize that his course may not have been challenging enough. We wish we had checked it out. If someone graduates from the same school as their sighted counterparts, well, that looks more impressive.

252

One of the women we hired spent an entire week, before starting work, practicing how she would get to the job. That kind of motivation is impressive, especially since the thing the manager in her department cares most about is absenteeism.

What didn't impress you about some of the applicants?

There was a sense of entitlement among the job candidates who didn't get hired. Their attitude was, You should give me a job because I'm blind.

The other turn-off is people who come in here and say, "I want to work for your company; I hear you hire blind people." That's ridiculous. Or they say, "I want to work for the telephone company." The manager at the phone company asks, "What do you want to do here, wash dishes?" And the answer is, "I'll do anything." That's the wrong answer.

Companies need people who can *fill specific job openings and demonstrate that they possess the specific skills to do the job.* We're not an assessment center.

Any other comments?

Just one more thought about the interview process. An employment manager once said, "If you get into an interview and they like you, and they think you could do the job, you'll probably get the job. If they like you, and think *maybe* you could do the job, you'll probably get it. But if they don't like you—even if they know you could do the job—you won't get it."

Personal chemistry makes or breaks the interview.

Interview with the Department Head
of a Word-Processing Division

Have you ever interviewed and hired a blind job applicant?

Yes, I was able to do so when I joined this company. I tried to bring a blind job applicant on board when I worked for another company, but there was resistance.

Why?

My boss was open, but he told me I was going to have a difficult time getting it through upper-level management because they were going to have to purchase a computer. Then I went to Personnel, and their objections were that they didn't know whether they could accommodate a blind person, whether they were going to have to change the elevators and put braille up all over the place. They started asking me job-accommodation questions I had no idea about. I hadn't thought of them. But they were interested in complying with the law, and they were also very interested in placing someone with me, figuring that if I had a successful candidate, I could get things started. But it had to be successful with me first.

So you went ahead?

Yes. Personnel knew they weren't in compliance with the suggested guidelines. They needed to do this work and they figured I could help them do it—comply with the law and get this set up. They knew it was coming. I was cautioned about the emotional aspects of it, because everybody has to buy into it, and then if it doesn't work out, it's devastating for everybody. I was probably more willing to go through with it because I had a woman who was mentally ill, a schizophrenic, and I had to terminate her. It wasn't the nicest thing I've ever done, but from that I had confidence that if someone couldn't do the job, I could say to them, "I'm sorry, it has nothing to do with your blindness; you can't do this job." So that was the one thing Personnel had an objection to. Was I strong enough to supervise them, or to possibly terminate somebody?

254

Then what?

Personnel put us through an awareness training, like what to say to a blind person. They showed us a movie during the lunch hour, so that all the employees in the entire company could drop in and watch. We even visited a local rehabilitation center for the blind.

So where did the resistance come from?

My boss's boss. He wasn't a risk-taker in any way. He was someone who lay low, didn't like attention; and if you're going to hire a blind person, you're going to get attention, and you *are* viewed as a risk-taker. Plus, the company started laying off people . . . it was going through difficulties. I left shortly after that.

How are things different in this company?

The people here, even the environment, are different. My boss and I are very compatible. The first thing he said, before he committed to anything, was that he wanted to talk to other managers who had hired blind workers. We attended a Project with Industry meeting. After that, he gave me the go-ahead: "Okay, it you're comfortable with it." He had seen a bunch of people who were comfortable with it.

How did you recruit blind candidates?

We went through Project with Industry, and they referred Sally. People already knew I was pursuing blind candidates. I was looked at as a do-gooder: "Oh, that's so nice of you!" That bothered me. Not everybody was so sociable; not everybody was as open. Then I started to get nervous: Maybe I'm going to make a fool of myself. So I asked for an awareness training that was different from the one at the previous company. It was run by a blind person from Project with Industry, and it was quite good. People got a chance to ask all the stupid things they wanted to ask, like "How is she going to get here?" "Does the dog have fleas?" "Can I pet the dog?" "Who is going to take the dog outside for a walk?" These are questions you want to ask, but can't during an interview. The only thing a supervisor can ask is "These are the hours. Are they a problem for you?" Supervisors need to be reassured somehow during the conversation that they don't have to worry about absenteeism or somebody constantly being late.

What impressed you about Sally?

Sally had already worked before, and had handled the job for three years. She had had the responsibility and had proven herself.

Would you have hired Sally without prior work experience?

Probably. You have to be very innovative to get people today. I've had co-op workers from high school, teenagers working while they were still in school on a two-thirds basis. And everybody thought that was awful, but it worked. I've recruited retired workers. I look for a good match. If someone can do that type of job, that's what I care about. I *do* care about people fitting in, and I worried about the teenagers fitting in with the older people, but that became less of a problem when people found out they had something in common—even if it was the job and they all hated me.

What were some of the concerns people had about Sally?

Lunch, going to the bathroom . . . the usual stuff.

Did these concerns come to light?

Not once she was here. One of the guys who had been pretty resistant got some work back from Sally, and there wasn't one error in it. He came and told me . . . said he wanted me to know. He's never told me anything positive about anybody else. He's always complaining. But he was very impressed. And he went over to her talking computer and asked her, "How does that thing work, anyway?" Now he's interested in the equipment. I know he thought it would never work out.

Has the company hired other blind workers?

Yes. A blind woman happened to come around and leave her resume. Elizabeth, in another department, hired her.

Do you think Sally paved the way for the second hire?

No question. Elizabeth has had a lot of turnover in her area, and some really hard times. She probably would not have been that much of a risk-taker if she hadn't known about my experience . . . if she hadn't been educated.

Do you think it's wise to mention one's blindness on a resume?

I don't think I would.

How would you have felt if Sally had applied for a position with you and you hadn't known before the interview that she was blind?

Okay . . . so what? I would have thought that it wasn't that important to her. You see, I'm used to surprises. I still get surprised when a man shows up for a position, since this has traditionally been a female-type job. And I get surprised when a black person shows up, too. I'm white, I think in white terms, and when I meet a black person, I'm surprised. I'm always surprised.

So you don't think blind applicants should have to disclose before the interview?

No. Has anybody ever called me up and said, "By the way, I'm black"? I'm a manager; I should be able to deal with any applicant who comes through my door. It might be more difficult for a new manager. If it's somebody who's been around for a while, at least three years, they're not going to be as concerned. Besides, if the candidate is being referred by Personnel, they are not coming unannounced.

Personnel generally does the prescreening. They're going to make a match mentally, in their heads. They would never send me anybody who comes in in jeans; they know me. And yet I watch somebody arriving on a bike be sent to another office.

The only advantage of mentioning it beforehand is that the shock value isn't there, so you don't put the employer at a disadvantage if *they* don't have the social graces to handle it.

Why can't they call just before they arrive, and say, "By the way . . . "? And make it "by the way"; you don't have to flash lights, just say, "By the way, I have a seeing-eye dog."

I hire minorities. I have Spanish-speaking people and two Indian women who work for me. I hire men in traditionally female positions. Personnel knows that about me. They know their managers, and they know the ones who hire minorities, and that would include someone who's blind.

What is the best point of entry into the company?

The way this company works is a bit different from most because we are made up of small satellite operations, so you should apply to the division in the location where you want to work. You don't have to go through Personnel. I advertise in the local papers, and people respond directly to me.

So, conceivably, a person could simply call up the receptionist in the location where they wanted to work, ask for the name of the hiring manager, and send a letter of application directly to that person?

Yes. Now, in the last company I worked for, you had to be prescreened by Personnel. It depends on the company.

Did any other issues surface?

My boss was concerned about somebody having to take Sally to lunch, or get her to work. He asked me a couple of times, "Now, you're not obliged to go pick her up or anything?" I said, "No! That's not up to me. However, if she gets the bus down to Route 2, we can let everybody know that she needs a ride up from Route 2." And he said, "Yeah, that's true! Yeah!" He liked that idea. But he didn't want me to hire somebody and then have them be my obligation after-hours.

258

Is there any other advice you would like to give to blind job seekers?

Yes. You know, semantics plays a large part in every conversation, but if they say the word "blind," then I can say the word "blind." I don't know why it's a difficult word to say; I don't know what's happened, that people don't want to say it. For some reason, it's hard to use the word in a sentence unless the blind person does first. Then you feel more comfortable: "Oh, my God! I can say it!"

So, you're saying that it's important for the blind job applicant to bring up the subject of blindness? If they say, "You must have questions about my blindness. Let's talk about it.", that would be a big relief?

Big. Don't you think so? The interviewer can't ask certain questions, like how they're going to get to work, because of hidden prejudices. So you can't ask, but you're dying to. Especially a person in Personnel, who's going to go to the line manager and say, "I've got this great candidate, but they're blind." "So how are they going to get here?" "I don't know; I can't ask, and you can't, either." "Yeah, but I've got to know."

Will Sally be as productive as her sighted counterparts?

We'll find out. We've just established company standards, which I have been pushing for. She will be measured just like everybody else. But I don't think Sally will have any trouble reaching and surpassing the goal.

* * * *

You now have some idea of what employers think. In the next chapter, we will look at strategies for dealing with employers' concerns. ¤

Chapter 6
Managing a
Successful Interview

They call it interview anxiety: That sense that your entire future rests on the results of one thirty- to sixty-minute performance—a performance that feels completely out of your control.

For the blind job seeker, the normal interview anxiety is heightened by other questions, like What kind of employer will I be meeting? Will the interviewer be able to get past my blindness to concentrate on my potential contributions to the company? Will I get an equal chance to compete for the job? Will I be aware of when the interviewer comes out of their office to meet me? Will my handshake be met with thin air? Will we have to walk across a thickly carpeted room where I won't hear the sound of the interviewer's footsteps? Will I crash into a coffee table or chair? Bottom line: Will I be able to perform at the critical moment and convey the right impression?

"It's not a matter of reducing stress," explained a seminar participant, "it's a matter of *managing* stress. When you go on a job interview, you have to find the right building, the front door, the room. By the time you get there, you're frazzled."

You are not alone.

The employers we interviewed confessed that they were *very* nervous about interviewing blind applicants. For most, it was the first blind person they had ever met. The unknown can be intimidating. As one employer put it, "Hiring people in general is risky, but hiring a blind job applicant appears even riskier."

Sitting across the desk from an otherwise qualified blind applicant, the employer is thinking: Will this candidate impose unnecessary demands on others? Will he need lots of expensive equipment that I have to provide? How will co-workers feel about working with a blind person? How independently will this blind employee move around the office or building complex? Will I be able to criticize this person for poor performance, and, heaven forbid, possibly even fire this blind person if things don't work out?

With real concerns on both sides of the desk—concerns which are often unspoken—it's a wonder the process works at all.

But it does.

Thousands of blind employees are testimony to the fact that you can learn to control these interview variables if you know how. In fact, because of the discomfort of many employers, you can control the interview by taking the initiative. This chapter will discuss specific strategies for preparing for and managing a successful interview.

PREPARING FOR THE INTERVIEW—MENTALLY

You have more control over the interview process than you think. To manage each interview opportunity successfully, you must prepare *mentally, physically,* and *strategically* for that all-important chance to prove you are the right person for the job. Here are some steps which will put you in the right frame of mind:

1. *Know What You Want, and Believe in Yourself*

If you *really* know what you want to do, if you believe you have the talent to do it, and if you really believe that your blindness will not stand in the way, then you have taken the first giant step toward getting what you want. A positive attitude is a necessity. One seminar participant put it this way:

"What is it you want? If you can answer that, you are halfway there. If people are clear about what they want, they generally can overcome the obstacles to get there.

"When you're dealing with corporate America, you're dealing with people who are not trained to look at some broader perspective. So, while you may be black, or white with a difference, or gay, or whatever, these folks are more comfortable dealing with the mainstream culture. The only way to get past this is to know what you want, and to go after it. No one else can do that work for you."

The opposite is also true.

If you don't know what you want, if you're not quite sure you can compete with your sighted peers, if you feel embarrassed using low-vision aids or braille, if you cringe at the thought of taking on something new, then you will always be victimized by the pre-interview jitters, which will have a negative effect on the employer.

Genuine self-confidence seems to come to those blind people who have benefited from an effective rehabilitation program, who understand the attitudes of the sighted public toward blindness, and who make an effort to mix with a wide range of blind people, to watch them, and to benefit from their experiences, mistakes, and winning strategies.

Qualifications alone will not win the job in most cases; it is the *general impression* you make during the interview that the hiring manager will remember long after you leave the office. If you are confident and in control of your job search, it will be obvious to others.

2. *Remember, Interviewing Is a Two-Way Street*

It always feels like the interviewer holds all the cards: You need a job, and the employer has the power to give it to you, or not. That's only half of the picture. In truth, the employer needs a good employee every bit as much as you need a good job. Treat the interview process as a mutually beneficial exchange.

While the employer's purpose is to evaluate your technical and interpersonal skills and your potential fit in the organization, *your* purpose is to evaluate the job responsibilities, the potential for advancement, the expectations of your supervisor and his or her management style, and whether the organization's climate is the right fit for you. You are also there to evaluate the position within the context of your career goals—now and in the future.

The same mutual analysis should take place regarding your disability. The employer wants to know how your blindness will affect your performance on the job. That's fair. And you want to know how the company's attitude toward blindness will affect you and your advancement in the company. Looking at the interview as a mutually beneficial exchange can help to alleviate some of the anxiety about the process.

3. *Go With the Flow . . . But Know Where You're Going*

A large number of hiring managers aren't well versed in the fine art of interviewing. A production manager may know his or her job inside out but be inept at interviewing job applicants. Add to this scenario the fact that most interviewers are nervous about your blindness and handicapped by their lack of experience in interviewing blind job applicants, and you can see that if you *are* adept at interviewing, if you *do* know what topics should be covered, if you *can* discuss job-related blindness issues skillfully, then you can be in the driver's seat.

The unskilled interviewer will be impressed and grateful, since you will make his or her job easier.

Take the case of Jeff McNaulty, who was interviewing for a position as a computer programmer. On his *third* interview with a prospective company, the interviewer was still not persuaded that a blind person could really be a programmer. So he asked Jeff, "What if we didn't hire you as a programmer, but found something else for you in the company?"

Jeff didn't hesitate: "I'm a good programmer, and programming is what I want to do. If I don't get the position here, I guess I'll keep looking." They hired him. This is a true story. The personnel manager explained why: "He knew what he wanted, and we were impressed by that."

4. *Understand Rejection As Part of the Process*

Rejection causes us to look inward, and that's okay—as long as you keep a healthy perspective on what rejection means.

Rejection may mean that the boss's niece needed a summer internship, not that you weren't qualified for the position. Rejection may mean that another candidate had knowledge of one additional piece of software, not that you couldn't handle the job. Rejection may mean that the interviewer had a bad day—the interview was "off" from the start. Rejection may mean that a pending layoff in another department forced an internal transfer of personnel into the position you wanted. You'll never know for sure, *so don't take rejection personally.*

It's part of the game.

Of course, rejection may also mean that you weren't qualified for the job. That does happen, after all. In any event, the odds are that you will be rejected many times before you land the job of your dreams. Here's how one seminar participant explained it:

"The whole job-search process is fraught with rejection, and I know many people who get done in by that process. They start believing everything they hear. The people who get past this are able to say, 'I'm hearing all this stuff, yet I'm going to keep the tension going by getting the job.' These people get all kinds of rejection, but they keep the tension in the process; they never stop, not even after a good interview."

5. *Keep a Perspective On the Labor Market*

The fewer job leads you have, and the fewer interviews you get, the more important each interview becomes in your mind. Each interview seems like the last opportunity: "If I don't get this one, it's all over. There won't be another chance like this one."

Nonsense.

We've said it before, and it's worth repeating: *The labor market in this country is so diverse, so dynamic and massive, that you should never fall into the trap of assuming that opportunities for employment are so limited.*

Although it is true that negative attitudes toward blindness will limit the number of interview opportunities you get, recognize that no matter how many times you miss out on your "dream job," another chance is right around the corner—literally. There are more job openings in this country every day than you could possibly apply for.

PREPARING FOR THE INTERVIEW—PHYSICALLY

Like it or not, the sighted world is obsessed with appearances. A well-groomed, impeccably dressed man or woman commands attention upon entering a room. The assumption is that this smartly attired person cares about him- or herself (self-respect) and doesn't mind letting other people know it (self-confidence). The "message" is an important one to convey to employers. Survey after survey concludes that employers rate appearance near the top of the list in evaluating candidates.

And just how fussy are these employers? Very. To be certain that you completely understand how judgmental the sighted world is about appearances, read these two articles that appeared in *The Wall Street Journal,* and remember the poor job applicant who was rejected because of his socks the next time you dress for an interview.

Businesswomen's Broader Latitude in Dress Codes Goes Just So Far
by Kathleen A. Hughes
The Wall Street Journal

"Clothes never shut up."
—from *Femininity,* by Susan Brownmiller

A decade ago, "The Woman's Dress for Success Book" propelled female executives into somber suits and blouses with big floppy bows at the neck. Then, a few years ago, a barrage of media stories reported that women had achieved enough success to look more feminine. It was fine to loosen up and wear dresses.

Now the miniskirt is back. The August issue of *Vanity Fair* magazine features a story entitled "Smart Women Wear Short Skirts," complete with a picture of Gloria Steinem, the editor of *Ms.* magazine and a renowned feminist, in one. The article, like others elsewhere, proclaims that "power women are hitching their hemlines inches above the knee."

Maybe so. But interviews with dozens of executives, both male and female, found that most would be shocked to see miniskirts on female executives. Indeed, the consensus seems to be that, despite the relaxation of dress codes, it still isn't acceptable to look too feminine—or too sexy or too cute—in corporate America.

Those interviewed say most female executives dress in a professional manner. But they can also recall vividly at least one inappropriate outfit that influenced their judgment of a woman's capability.

Signaling Weakness

"Looking extremely feminine gives the message that you need to be taken care of," says Brenda York, president of the Academy of Fashion and Image Consultants in McLean, Va. "It says you aren't as serious as someone who would refrain from dressing like that."

Consider Joe O. Swain, vice president of auditing at Rainier Bancorp. in Seattle. Mr. Swain says he recently stopped by the office of a female manager at the company and found her wearing a dress with a "really bright blue background with really large flowers with pink petals and bright yellow in the center." The low-cut dress had short sleeves, he adds, and when the woman moved her arms, "you could see the underarm."

That dress bothered him. "I thought, Well that's a very loud and inappropriate dress," he says. "I began to question her competence."

Not surprisingly, the issue strikes some feminists as absurd. "It's a big waste of time to stand in front of your closet and worry about whether someone will think badly of you because of a lacy collar," says Letty Cottin Pogrebin, a founding editor of *Ms.* "It's a terrible duality. It has nothing to do with our performance."

Still, in actual practice the results of such readings can be dire. John T. Molloy, who wrote a "Dress for Success" book for men as well as the one for women, says that as part of a study he asked the managers of about 10,000 female office workers to describe the women's style of dress. Then he tracked the women's career progress over three years.

He found that the female executives whose attire was described as "extremely feminine" were typically paid less and promoted less frequently. The highest-paid women, on the other hand, were those whose dress was described as professional, dull, conservative, non-sexy or non-frilly. Women whose clothes were termed conservative or traditional were twice as likely to receive promotions as those whose dress was labeled frilly or frivolous, or occasionally frilly or occasionally sexy.

"If you wear very fluffy or sexy clothing or a miniskirt," Mr. Molloy asserts, "you are cutting short not only your skirt but your career."

Dress and Success
Women in sales positions whose attire is described as conservative by their managers outperform their colleagues. A breakdown:

	DRESS			
JOB PERFORMANCE	VERY PROFESSIONAL AND VERY CONSERVATIVE	APPROPRIATE	SEXY: FRILLY OR FASHIONABLE	POORLY DRESSED
Top performers	12.5%	12.6%	11.5%	1.9%
Consistently above average	60.9	41.1	31.0	30.8
Average or below	21.9	44.2	54.0	50.0
Failing	4.7	2.1	3.4	17.3

Source: Survey by John T. Molloy of 298 women in corporate sales positions.

Men also pay for sartorial mistakes. Though the uniform nature of men's suits provides fewer opportunities for dramatic gaffes, and men rarely have to worry about sexist responses, they are often judged harshly for looking too sloppy, too casual, too quirky or too flashy. As with women, such infractions lead some executives to question their judgment and business acumen. (See accompanying story.)

While the executives interviewed agree that it's certainly possible to look both feminine and professional, just what it means to look "too feminine" is open to debate. When the executives were asked to cite specific outfits they find inappropriate, their opinions varied by industry. But both men and women mentioned outfits that were too flowery, too tight, too short, too low-cut, too "cutesy" or too loud. They also complained about spike heels, hats, and excessive makeup and jewelry.

Dress consultants and some female executives provide a more detailed list of sartorial offenses in the office, including sleeveless dresses, scoop backs, colored stockings and, in such industries as investment banking, pastel or pink outfits.

"Pink and pastel shades give off messages of being very fragile and very feminine," says Ms. York, the dress consultant. "Those colors don't have the power that neutral colors have, such as black, navy or gray."

Ms. York points out, however, that flowery dresses may be suitable in "public relations, advertising and fashion fields." She says that "if flowery (materials) are in vogue, it's expected" that female executives in those industries wear them.

The executives queried agree that the biggest clothing mistakes seem to show up on job applicants and other visitors from outside an office. A female candidate for a job involving labor negotiation at a large Los Angeles savings-and-loan association arrived in a blue and pink flowery dress with "little flouncy sleeves" and a "little lace collar," says Patricia Benninger, a vice president of human resources there.

The dress "turned off all the credibility she could have built up during the interview," says Ms. Benninger. "My feelings were, She doesn't know the job." The outfit, she adds, said that the woman was "someone who could be easily persuaded," and that "this person couldn't stand up to toughness."

Some executives conclude that if a woman wears an inappropriate outfit to a job interview she probably doesn't understand the realities of the business world—and thus isn't a suitable candidate. Carl J. Sette, vice president and resident manager of E.F. Hutton & Co. in Stockton, Calif., says that a woman applying for an account-executive position showed up in a low-cut blue and white paisley dress that also featured a slit in the skirt.

Mr. Sette, who had talked to this woman on the phone, determined she was well qualified, and formed a good impression, turned her down after meeting with her. "It bothers me when people try to advertise (physical) assets," says Mr. Sette. "Instead of looking at an equal professional, you start questioning."

Most of the executives surveyed say they haven't seen many miniskirts on female executives yet, and those who have seem to be concentrated in the entertainment industry. Richard Leary, vice president of advertising and publicity at Taft Entertainment Co. in Los Angeles, says he has seen a few in the company's legal-affairs and music divisions. "My honest feeling is that it's a little distracting," he says, adding, "In some cases, it's as inappropriate as a man wearing shorts."

Seeming 'the Little Girl'

Sexual signals aren't the only ones miniskirts may give off. "A short skirt casts you in the role of the little girl, and we don't take little girls seriously in the workplace," says Virginia O'Leary, a visiting scholar at Radcliffe College and the author of a recent study of female bosses.

If looking too feminine or sexy isn't likely to advance one's career, neither is looking too cute. And it's usually the youngest members of an office who unwittingly fall into a cuteness trap, executives say.

Nan Tepper, the director of personnel at CBS Inc. in Los Angeles, recalls a young female researcher who sometimes wore socks with polka dots, longish shorts and cotton shirts with a bow tie. The woman had complained to her that she wasn't being promoted. "It hasn't dawned on some younger women that to be taken seriously as a professional you have to present the image," says Ms. Tepper.

While most female executives say they rule out wearing "cute" outfits to work, some confess to slipping occasionally. Terry L. Flett, a Los Angeles lawyer, says she recently wore a blue sweater with a white lace collar and a green tartan skirt to her office. Two of the firm's partners and several secretaries, she says, told her she looked cute. She never wore the outfit to work again. "Cute seems to be the opposite of serious," she says.

Suitable Alternatives

Such experiences don't mean a dark suit is the only safe bet. When asked to describe professional dress for women, most executives also mention tailored dresses and skirts worn with a jacket. Moreover, the frequency of suit wearing seems to be down. In a study of some 1,300 women in corporate sales positions, Mr. Molloy, the author, found that about 50% of those studied wear suits two or three days a week now, compared with 70% five years ago.

In fact, many executives say that the classic man-tailored suit now looks dated on women. Some even find it comical.

Lawrence W. Farmer, an executive vice president of Weyerhaeuser Mortgage Co. in Woodland Hills Calif., hired an executive recruiter after talking to her on the phone. She arrived at work wearing a very conservative heavy blue suit, practical shoes and a little bow tie made from a blue, green and black plaid material. She was carrying a brand-new briefcase.

"She looked like she was going right through the manual of how you do this," says Mr. Farmer. "I thought she looked a little funny. She looked uncomfortable." ¤

Male Executives Also Suffer
For Their Sartorial Mistakes
by Kathleen A. Hughes
The Wall Street Journal

Men are rarely accused of looking too masculine at work, partly because in the male-dominated business world it's almost impossible to look *too* masculine.

But the safe haven of a suit doesn't prevent men from making sartorial gaffes, and such transgressions are often noted by employers or potential employers with consequences as serious as those for women.

Most of the executives interviewed claim they don't pay much attention to how expensive a suit looks or whether it conforms to the latest fashion, unless it's extremely outdated. But they say they do frequently take note of ill-fitting suits, unironed shirts, ties that are too short and tacky tie clips, as well as socks and shoes that don't convey a professional image.

"The biggest mistake is not fitting in or wearing something that says 'blue collar,'" says John T. Molloy, the author of the "Dress for Success" books. "Those who know the rules will look disparagingly at someone who doesn't follow them."

Baring the Pocket Protector

Consider the hapless applicant for a $150,000-a-year position as a vice president and general manager of a large Midwestern company. Gary Silverman, a regional managing director of Korn/Ferry International, an executive-recruiting firm, had sent the candidate over for an interview with the company's top brass.

"The client mentioned the fellow had taken off his suit jacket and had on a short-sleeve shirt with a pocket protector," Mr. Silverman recalls. "He said (the applicant) just wouldn't fit in when standing up in front of the directors and making a presentation."

However, donning a classic conservative suit isn't always a guarantee of safety, as the rules vary with different industries. "In the entertainment industry, if you wear a pin-stripe suit they may be suspicious of you," says David Handelman, senior vice president and general counsel of Twentieth Century Fox Film Corp.

There are geographical differences as well. Mr. Silverman says that when he interviews in Arkansas or Georgia he isn't surprised to find male job applicants wearing lime-green or powder-blue polyester suits, patent leather shoes and white belts. "I presume that's acceptable there," he says. "But clearly in the Midwest, the East or the West it isn't acceptable."

Whatever their color, ill-fitting clothes are an obvious drawback, particularly when the fit is way off. Phillip Humphries, the employment manager at Chevron Corp. in San Francisco, recalls one over-weight applicant on a college campus who showed up wearing a light-colored suit that was "probably four sizes too small."

"Everything bulged," says Mr. Humphries. "The buttons were almost popping off, and the suit looked like it was held together with steel bands." The man wasn't hired for an engineering position despite a "fairly good" academic record, he notes, adding that the suit wasn't the only reason the candidate was turned down. "He was lacking in self-confidence," Mr. Humphries explains, "and he had some nervous mannerisms."

Looking too fashionable can also be a problem. "The men who run America run it blue, gray and dull," says Mr. Molloy. "If you try to spruce up the look, you're in trouble."

One of the most serious offenses seems to be unprofessional footwear. Among the items likely to raise eyebrows are socks that are white, beige, brightly colored or large-patterned, as well as sloppy shoes, saddle shoes and lounge slippers.

Suede Slip-ons

Martha Heiberg, director of personnel at Ticor Title Insurance Co. in Los Angeles, says one man applying for a job made the mistake of wearing suede slip-on shoes. "The two people who talked to him said, 'I couldn't hire him because he was wearing bedroom slippers,'" she says. "They liked him otherwise."

He isn't the only one to suffer for the wrong footwear at Ticor. Noreen Brown, the company's employment manager, says last year a young man applied unsuccessfully for a position as a methods analyst. He came to the interview wearing a sport coat, pants and maroon argyle socks.

"He was fine," Ms. Brown explains. "It was the manager that didn't like his socks. The manager thought the guy was weird because of his socks."

Socks have also been an issue at Price Waterhouse in Los Angeles. "I've seen beige socks and been repulsed by them," says Merle Hopkins, an area director of recruitment and continuing education for the accounting firm. The wrong attire, he notes, "commands attention and therefore distracts from what may be a very important discussion." ¤

There are hundreds of books, magazine articles, and pamphlets that will tell you how to dress for an interview. Read a few. What we want to emphasize in this book is the fact that interview etiquette is *doubly* important for the blind job seeker. Why? Because blindness will play such a large role in the interview, you can't afford to lose points over things you can control. Because most sighted people don't expect people who are blind to be snappy dressers; they think it's strictly a visual phenomenon. The minute you break down one stereotype, in the minds of sighted employers, you open their minds to other possibilities. It jogs their prejudices.

Here are a few pointers:

¤ Dress codes vary only a little from one office environment to another. A safe rule of thumb is to wear a conservative (but stylish) suit.
¤ Too much of anything is out—too much perfume, cologne, makeup, jewelry, hair, beard, etc.
¤ Proper attire includes good grooming, so if you have been puttering in the garden, get a manicure. Make sure your clothes are lint-free and pressed, and your shoes polished.

There are few things that are more impressive to a sighted person than a blind person who is impeccably and stylishly dressed. People just don't expect it.

That doesn't mean that the right outfit will compensate for a lack of technical competence and interpersonal skills, but a well-dressed applicant makes a positive first impression, which gets you started on the right foot.

PREPARING FOR THE
INTERVIEW—STRATEGICALLY

All of the skills you need to conduct a successful interview can be learned. Read up on the subject and practice, practice, practice. Stage mock interviews with friends and relatives, and sign up for an interview-skills workshop offered through your local community college or YWCA. The more prepared you are, the more self-assured you will be during the interview. Here are a few things you can do to prepare:

1. *Eradicate Painful Speech Patterns and Study Body Language*

Tape a few mock interview sessions and listen to yourself. How many times did you say "you know"? Poor grammar and sloppy speech habits offend many interviewers who care not only about what potential recruits have to say, but *how* they say it. Eradicate painful speech patterns, like constant hemming and hawing, overused phrases like "moving right along," "that's for sure," and faddish words, like "awesome."

What about your body language? Ask for some feedback from a trusted friend. Are you stiff and uptight, or loose and natural? If you are partially sighted, videotape your interview rehearsals and correct any negative body language, such as slumping shoulders, fidgeting hands, rocking, and absence of eye contact.

2. *Treat Each Interview As a Unique Opportunity*

Each interview must be prepared for individually. That means conducting a thorough research of the company and the job—and don't forget the importance of networking as a means of obtaining that information.

"The major reason that most candidates do not receive job offers is that they neglect to prepare thoroughly for each interview," says Jack Erdlen in his book CAREERSEARCH.

"Many qualified applicants are rejected because they fail to do their homework.

"In most interview circumstances, the candidate has been prescreened through a resume or telephone conversation, and the meeting with the employer becomes the critical factor in the job-hunting process. Most job hunters overlook the importance of tailoring their presentation for every job interview. Job seekers must take the time to prepare for each individual interview."

Investigate the details of the job to the point where you can describe the alternative techniques you will use to compensate for your blindness. Remember, you are there to lighten the load for your prospective boss.

Be ready to answer the request "Tell me about yourself." Prepare a fluent, spontaneous-sounding three-to-five minute oral presentation about your experiences, skills, accomplishments, and goals, and how these relate *specifically* to the job at hand. Hiring managers are looking for a good match between the demands of the job and the skills of prospective job applicants. You can identify that match in the interview to your advantage.

3. *Be Knowledgeable About Reasonable Accommodations*

It's your job to know about accommodations that can be made which will enable you to be as productive as your sighted counterparts. You cannot expect employers to be versed in this area.

Be prepared to talk about the types of adaptations other blind people are using on the job (consult The Job Index or Job Opportunities for the Blind). This includes non-technical job adaptations, such as readers, drivers, braille or recording services, and so forth. Consider beforehand whether you can pay for these resources yourself, and how many hours you will need them. Think through the possible complications. For example, if the job involves travel by car, will your assistants be able to drive you, even on short notice? Have the facts ready to present to the now-attentive interviewer. This is the way to convince a reluctant employer that you are a problem solver.

4. Be Ready for the Next Call

Have your braille slate or cassette recorder near the phone and ready to go when the next interviewer calls. You will be prepared and in control.

Be sure to ask for the correct spelling of his or her name. Don't ask for directions to get there. Give the impression that getting places, for you, is no big deal. Later, you can call the organization's switchboard and ask the operator for specific directions.

5. Do a Dry Run

Why mess up a precious interview opportunity simply because you didn't allow enough time to get there, took the wrong bus, or otherwise got off to a bad start? Reduce your pre-interview jitters by making a dry-run trip to the place of the interview. Familiarize yourself with the route, the building, and the specific office and floor where you will be meeting with a prospective boss. You will be glad you did on the day of the interview.

THE BIG DAY HAS ARRIVED

Allow yourself plenty of time to get there. Arriving early gives you a chance to catch your breath and relax . . . well, try.

If you are delayed by more than five minutes, call. Keeping the boss informed about possible project delays is an important business trait; why not plant this characteristic in the prospective employer's mind about you?

In most cases, the security guard or receptionist will call the office of the interviewer to announce your arrival. Typically, the interviewer's secretary will come out to greet you and escort you to the interviewer's office. This isn't because you are blind; it's a common courtesy extended to most guests.

If the interviewer does not send out his or her secretary to escort you to the right office, ask confidently and politely for directions, or, if you need more assistance, for someone to accompany you. Don't feel compelled to demonstrate what a great traveler you are, if doing so will cause you added stress and lessen your poise. Since you want to arrive at the interviewer's office with as little fanfare as possible, simply tell your sighted escort exactly what kind of help you need, *e.g.,* "I can follow behind you" or "May I take your arm?"

The more difficult situation to handle is when they send a security guard to escort you, implying that you are a safety risk! Try to avoid this situation, but don't do battle with the security guard and cause a scene. Your primary concern is to get to the interviewer's office on time and without causing a commotion. Don't sweat the small stuff.

Once you reach the proper office, the secretary or receptionist may invite you to sit down until the interviewer is ready to see you. This is another chance to sell yourself. Secretaries, especially those close to their bosses, often remark on particular candidates who strike them as exceptional (exceptionally good or exceptionally bad). A secretary who says "I really liked so-and-so" adds a few points to that person's interview rating. Likewise, even a brief comment, like "Boy, was that so-and-so weird" is likely to cancel out a candidate, or at least put a question mark in the mind of the interviewer.

Refrain from smoking while you wait, and politely decline coffee or tea. Pre-interview jitters can lead to an accidental spill on that spotless interview suit.

Do allow the secretary to take your hat and coat; sitting there with your coat on when the interviewer comes out to greet you looks like you're already on your way out! Position yourself in the chair or sofa in such a way that as soon as the interviewer comes out to greet you, you can rise crisply from your seat and move forward to shake his or her hand firmly (a limp handshake connotes a limp personality).

Researchers say that most employers make up their minds about job applicants in the *first four minutes.* That means *every minute counts,* from the moment you stand up to greet the interviewer and shake hands, to the next few minutes as you settle into a designated chair and participate in some small talk. You are smiling, friendly, relaxed. If you're dealing with the shock factor, you will have to quickly finesse the interviewer's discomfort with some reassuring words, like "Thank you for taking the time to interview me."

Most interviewers start off with a bit of small talk. The two most common topics are the weather and sports. This small talk is important. This is part of those critical first few minutes, where you are establishing rapport with a total stranger. Plus, as a blind job applicant, you need to reassure your potential employer that you know what's going on around you, that you are informed, and that you can hold your own in any business-related social function—that blindness is neither a mental nor social handicap.

If you are applying for a sales or public relations position, you may find that the interview is conducted in an informal social setting, over lunch or breakfast at a nearby restaurant. This isn't simply a matter of fitting you into a tight schedule; it's intentional. Your social etiquette skills are being tested.

Steer clear of alcohol. Even if the interviewer orders a drink, you need a clear head. If you don't have enough sight to read the menu, be reasonable. Ask your host to read the main headings from the menu, and make your selection quickly. (By the way, have you had your table manners critiqued lately? As obnoxious as it is for a blind person to listen to sighted people chomp and slurp their way through a meal, it is equally distasteful for a sighted person to watch a blind person eat with poor table manners.) Here is your chance to show a prospective boss how well you handle yourself in a social setting.

This brings up another point.

There are occasions when the need to demonstrate your independence may not be as important as the need to be efficient. For example, if you and your prospective employer are zigzagging through a crowded restaurant on your way to a table for a luncheon interview, in a room strewn with armchairs, sofas, and coffee tables, it is simply more efficient to ask your interviewer for his or her arm to guide you across the room. Demonstrate that you are in control of whatever situation you are in, that you are aware of your surroundings, and that you are flexible enough to make things work. *All of us are dependent on someone else in certain situations.* Sighted people, too.

MANAGING THE INTERVIEW

No two interviews are alike.

Bringing together two unique individuals in an emotionally charged situation results in a personal chemistry with a life of its own. It is this chemistry—good or bad—that ultimately influences the outcome. The good news is, there are specific things you can do to strengthen this fragile relationship and improve the chemistry.

Here are some tips:

1. *Be Prepared for Different Interviewing Styles*

Most hiring managers structure interviews around their personal style of interaction, which varies from conversational to rigid fact-finding. A format many interviewers follow is to verify the "facts" presented on your resume before moving into general questions that test, among other things, your intelligence, capacity for honest self-analysis, human sensitivity, poise, and strength of character.

Occasionally you will run into an interviewer who skips the formalities altogether and focuses on your general attitude toward work and your philosophy of life. The assumption is, if your temperament and intelligence are good, you can learn the details of the job once you're on board.

If you interview with a large company, you will probably be prescreened by someone in Personnel who will make sure that you have the basic qualifications and don't exhibit any offensive personality or appearance traits. A savvy personnel manager also knows what kind of person Sam Cook likes down in Sales, or the fact that Martha Roberts doesn't like long hair.

Sometimes you will find yourself sitting across the table from a small army of interviewers—this is the so-called "search committee," or group interview. Here you will be fielding questions from hiring managers, co-workers, and possibly even members of the board of directors.

It is your job, during the interview, to assess the type and style of interview being conducted and to be responsive. If you have a good grasp of the topics which must be covered in any successful interview, then you are in control regardless of the interview style.

2. Don't Be Afraid to Take the Initiative

There will be times when it behooves you to take the initiative during the interview. Let's say you haven't properly researched the company. Early in the interview, you might say, "I wonder if you could give me some basic information about the job, the organization, and the people I might be working with. That way, I will be able to give you more helpful information about myself." (Know, however, that a skilled interviewer will be wondering why you don't know these things prior to the interview.)

If you quickly establish a good rapport with the interviewer, you might ask for a brief tour around the plant. Most "hot prospects" are given a tour of the workplace somewhere between the first interview and the actual job offer. The purpose of the guided tour is to show the plant off to a prospective employee, and to give the other workers a chance to meet candidates who are being considered for the position.

On-site tours are a great opportunity to get a feel for the environment, for management's rapport with the workers, and for the actual working conditions of the plant. It also gives you a chance to meet prospective co-workers.

Unfortunately, some employers will be reluctant to give you a tour, either because they are concerned about your mobility, or because they haven't "warned" the staff about your blindness. Encourage the interviewer to give you a tour as well. Why? For four good reasons:

- because as you chat easily with others, you demonstrate that you are capable of making those around you feel comfortable;
- because as you "talk shop" with workers, you demonstrate that you speak the language of the workplace, that you can make yourself understood, and that you know what you're talking about;
- because as you come across a piece of equipment—a computer terminal, typewriter, welding machine—which you would be expected to operate, and you say in a casual way, "Let me take a quick look at this . . .," or "Why don't I just make sure this is the type of equipment I'm familiar with. . . ," you demonstrate that you can operate it;
- because as you stroll down the corridor or weave around workbenches, you demonstrate that you are mobile.

Your unspoken message to prospective employers and co-workers is clear: you feel right at home.

3. *Personalize Your References*

Many employers discount references because, after all, they are given by people who were hand-picked by you, and because most references say only positive things. Nevertheless, the absence of good references speaks volumes. And, in your case, verification of your expertise, competence, work ethic, and overall personality to a resistant employer is highly desirable.

Always let your references know the specific job and company where you are applying for work. You are asking them to be available to respond over the phone to a hiring manager. By being kept informed, they can tailor their responses specifically to the job.

4. *Persuade by Example*

Here's the situation: The hiring manager sitting across the desk from you is impressed by your appearance, your credentials, and the way in which you conduct yourself during the interview. Still, your blindness is an "unknown" factor in the equation, which still makes the situation risky. How can you reduce the risk factor?

Try this. Hiring managers who are afraid to risk the unknown and employ a blind person are most likely to be persuaded to do so *by other hiring managers*—their counterparts in other organizations—who have successfully employed one or more blind employees. If one employer takes the plunge into uncharted waters and survives to talk about it, others will be less hesitant to follow in their wake.

Use this strategy carefully. You want to identify two or three blind individuals who you know are working successfully in a comparable position. The key words are *working successfully.* Don't tie your star to one that isn't shining.

Get to know these people. If you followed the job-search strategies outlined earlier in this book, you already know several blind individuals working in your field of interest. If not, contact the Job Opportunities for the Blind Project, the Job Index, or the Job Accommodation Network (JAN). JAN serves the employer community primarily as a consultant on specific employment-related accommodations, but they can also refer hesitant employers to experienced employers of people with disabilities, for general support.

Explain how their success could help you convince a reluctant employer to give you a chance. Ask the employees to ask their supervisors if they would be willing to talk to prospective employers about how blind workers manage on the job. Assure them that this would not involve a lot of time, simply a phone call or two, or perhaps a brief on-site visit.

This can be a highly effective strategy. Employers will ask other employers questions they are afraid to ask you directly. They can voice their fears and concerns with a peer and get the kind of response which will move them from "I just don't believe it can be done by a blind person" to "Oh, I see. That's how they do it."

5. *A Far-Out Approach for the Gutsy Job Seeker*

On October 19, 1987, when the stock market took a nosedive, senior managers at Merrill Lynch appeared on company video screens around the country to assure their account executives of the future stability of the stock market. And when Robert E. Allen was elected chairman of the board at AT&T, he introduced himself to employees on video within an hour of his selection.

Video communication has become a fixed asset in the business world. According to an article in *The New York Times,* American corporations will spend billions of dollars on video productions this year, some even sporting their own in-house television networks.

So what can this mean for you? Why not join the video craze and show employers exactly how blind individuals function independently? Most employers get stuck on the notion that a person simply cannot work productively without sight, no matter how qualified that person is. Because they do not know other blind people, and because they have not observed, first-hand, how various adaptations work, they cannot believe that braille, canes, dogs, talking computers, and the like actually assist a blind person in functioning well in a work environment.

One way to bring a disbelieving employer around is to demonstrate "live" just how you do perform certain tasks and move around. Here's how it works:

1. Ask friends and relatives if they own a camcorder—that is, a video camera with video recording equipment. If not, you can rent one.

2. Recruit a friend or relative to serve as your camera operator and co-producer. Don't let them shy away from the assignment because they lack experience. You only need a run-of-the-mill amateur home-movie maker.

3. Prepare a list of activities—both work-related and not—that demonstrate that you can work cooperatively and competitively. Broaden the scope of your "film" to include activities that show you leading a full, varied, and satisfying life. For example, you might prepare three lists of activities: one which is work-related, a second which focuses on volunteer activities, and a third which highlights your social life. List the activities in a storyline progression, so they follow one another logically. Now you are ready to shoot.

4. Why not start with an outdoor sequence? Ask the operator to film you walking out of your home, traveling several blocks, crossing a busy intersection, moving through revolving doors (your bank, perhaps), riding up escalators (at the mall), standing in line (at the post office), using an automated bank teller, boarding a crowded bus, shopping at the local market,

using the subway, picking up a sighted friend for coffee, getting off an elevator (at your favorite restaurant), working out at your health club, swimming in a crowded pool, hailing a cab to the airport, checking in at the airport and asking for gate directions, taking your children to the park, accompanying a frail grandparent to the doctor's office, going to the movies with a spouse . . . you've got the idea. Clearly, the purpose is to show employers that you lead a normal life, like anyone else. They may have assumed that you lived a lonely existence "in a world of darkness."

If you are employed, videotape yourself on the job (tell your boss you are preparing a video presentation on employment of the blind—well, that's true, isn't it?). If not, shoot scenes of yourself using the skills you want to sell, like operating a computer at home, conducting a meeting, lobbying legislators on the phone, dictating memos to a secretary, working with readers, etc. Take as many *action* shots as you can.

Finally, shoot a sequence of vignettes at home, doing ordinary everyday activities like vacuuming, laundry, dinner, feeding the baby, home maintenance, and so forth. Although these activities are not work-related, scenes of this kind broaden a sighted person's perspective of your lifestyle, and demonstrate your self-sufficiency.

5. The final step is to edit the tape. This is a highly discretionary process, as film editors will attest, but here are a few pointers.

Include in the final product only the best *few seconds* of each activity, and discard the rest. Most people's attention span is short. Employment-related shots should carry more weight, especially those shots that demonstrate your job-related skills. If you are applying for a job that requires extensive travel, for instance, focus on mobility shots. The entire video should not exceed 10 minutes in length.

Once you have edited the video portion, slip the tape into a VCR so you can dub an audio commentary to go along with it.

Standing at a curb, waiting to cross a busy intersection, your commentary might say: "Now I am paying attention to the direction of traffic flow. As soon as I hear the cars moving forward, I know that the lights have changed and I can begin to cross."

6. Make several copies of the video, and then borrow, rent, or buy one of the new portable videocassette players, which are about the size of a briefcase. Learn how to slip the cassette in and out easily and quickly.

7. Take your "live" demonstration with you to the next interview. Don't use it until you have already described your professional experience, education, technical skills, and interests as they relate to the job. Then, when the discussion turns to your blindness, be very sensitive to the employer's reactions, questions, and intonation. Does he or she really believe that you would be able to handle the job without sight? Is there still a nagging doubt in his or her mind? Would the employer benefit from actually seeing you in action? If the answer is yes, then you might say, "Look, I have a feeling that you still have a few doubts about my ability to be competitive with my co-workers. If I were in your position, I might have some doubts myself. Anyway, I've brought along a videotape which may help convince you that I am capable of handling this job. Why don't I just take a few minutes and show it to you?"

Then, place the videocassette player on the desk, in front of the interviewer, dim the lights, raise the curtain, and let the show begin.

Why Is This a Good Strategy?

This strategy shows the prospective employer that you are creative, able to work in a visual medium, considerate enough to meet their needs, and a person of action. Better yet, it educates the employer about how blind workers can function independently.

Since you may be interviewing with someone in Personnel instead of with a hiring manager at this point, offer to leave the cassette for the interviewer to share with others. This gives you a good excuse to phone several days later, to inquire about the return of the video. Your *real* intention, of course, is to maintain contact, express your enthusiasm for the job, and clarify any questions they may have about your candidacy.

Using a video in the job interview is another tool to break down the resistance many employers have toward hiring a blind employee. **Note:** As far as we know, this video strategy has never been tried. We present it as an idea, hoping someone will try it and let us know how it works.

FOUR ESSENTIAL QUALITIES EMPLOYERS LOOK FOR

Basically, all employers are looking for four essential qualities in the candidates they interview and eventually hire: (1) technical knowledge, (2) competence, (3) a strong work ethic, and (4) likeability. Your job, during the interview, is to demonstrate that you possess all four. Here's how:

1. *Technical Knowledge*

Early in the interview, you should spell out, *specifically,* the technical knowledge and skills that you possess relevant to the job. If you have a solid work history and good employer references, plus a record of accomplishments in your field, this should be easy. If not, bring actual samples of your work, as mentioned in Chapter 3. Letters of recommendation can also verify your expertise in a given field. If you are planning to work on a computer, bring in your laptop and give an on-site demonstration of how you use one of the more popular programs.

2. *Competence*

Competence has to do with using your technical knowledge to get things done. A competent person shows *results.* You may have a Ph.D. in theater arts, but if you can't work with people, aren't organized enough to stage events, or can't cope with major donors, then you are not competent on the job. Competent people make things happen.

That's why it's important, during the interview, to not limit your discussion to past job titles and duties, but to focus on *measurable accomplishments.* If you managed 100 theater prima donnas, organized over 200 stage plays, and raised $1,000,000 for theater repairs, then describe how you did it.

If you do not have work experience, use volunteer activities in the same way. If you are the legislative chairperson of a local chapter of a national organization of the blind, describe a lobbying campaign which you spearheaded. What was the *problem?* Insurance companies in your state were discriminating in the sale of insurance policies, on grounds of blindness. What *actions* did you take, and why? You held a legislative breakfast, to press members of your state senate and assembly to pass legislation which would prohibit such discrimination. You selected a site, set a date, sent invitations, prepared a list of exciting speakers, ordered the food, and pulled off the whole event. What were the *results?* Two key legislators immediately announced their intention to introduce a bill which would remedy the problem. Problem, action, results—these spell competence.

3. *A Strong Work Ethic*

Employers complain a lot these days that employees don't care about their work. In fact, most managers will tell you that poor performance in the workplace is the result of apathy, not incompetence or lack of knowledge. The successful companies Tom Peters identified in his best-selling book *In Search of*

Excellence were those which did motivate their employees to care about their jobs.

So how do you convince a prospective employer that you care? By sitting up straight in the interview and leaning ever so slightly toward the interviewer, and by listening intently to questions and responding with energy and enthusiasm. Don't be afraid to show how excited you are about the job. Enthusiasm is contagious and appreciated.

We're not suggesting that you burst into the interview room with all guns blazing, storm the interviewer's desk, and gush all over, but we are recommending that you be positive, alert, and responsive. When you speak, speak with confidence.

4. *Likeability*

The personal chemistry that develops between you and the interviewer will be the deciding factor in winning the interview. "Good vibes" are critical to all successful work environments and relationships.

Some people think, erroneously, that personal chemistry either happens or it doesn't—that nothing can be done to improve the interaction between two individuals. Wrong. How important to you was it to impress the girl who sat in back of you in geometry? And didn't you impress her mother (now your mother-in-law) twenty years later when you had to? We are all constantly trying to influence different people in our lives who are important to us.

You can break the ice quickly by sporting a smile. If you have prepared for the interview, you will feel more at ease about participating in the obligatory small talk that sets the tone of the interview. Don't be afraid to release your sense of humor, which is an effective quality in any job candidate. Most important, personal chemistry will be enhanced by your own natural curiosity and your sincere interest in the job, your prospective boss, and the company. People who demonstrate genuine interest in others seem to have a charismatic quality about them.

Don't be shy about asking your prospective boss about his or her supervisory style: "How do you communicate your performance expectations to your subordinates? How do your subordinates know when they've done a good job? Are you a 'meeting person', or do you tend to communicate by memo?" By showing sincere interest in the style and substance of your prospective boss, you will increase your likeability rating.

A FIFTH ESSENTIAL QUALITY FOR THE BLIND JOB CANDIDATE

There is one more quality that employers want to see in *blind* job applicants: self-sufficiency. Employers fear that bringing a blind applicant on board could mean more work for everyone—even though they're not about to say so during the interview.

Here's what a few seminar participants said:

"I was a personnel director, so I've been on both sides of the desk. You can 'feel' the difference between an applicant who will take charge of a problem, go with it, solve it, and alleviate the situation, and someone who is going to sit back and expect someone else to do it. It's that feeling of self-sufficiency that comes across in the interview."

* * * *

"I have found that the successful interviews I have had got around to a discussion of exactly how I would perform the job tasks. I didn't promise that I could do everything—I said I'd need help with some things—but I had thought through how I was going to do the job."

* * * *

"No matter what, you have to present yourself as a person who will contribute to the organization—not someone who will add to their workload or whatever problems they already have. You must use the job interview to gather information about the job to see how you are going to solve certain problems, and be able to present solutions to the employer."

One thing is certain: *Never end an interview without having an open and honest exchange about your blindness and your personal solutions to work-related problems.* If you don't, you can be certain that you are not seriously being considered for the job. Here are some points to get across:

1. You are a problem solver, not a problem creator. Years of dealing with your blindness have forced you to become a highly adaptable person who is accustomed to drawing upon your creativity and imagination to solve specific problems.
2. You will not use your blindness as an excuse for not carrying your share of the workload.
3. You are fully aware of the attitudinal barriers which can be created by your blindness, but you are well equipped to make people around you comfortable in your presence.

Your ability to discuss job-related blindness issues will be one of the most important tasks you face in the interview—some employers might say *the* most. Let's look at strategies for handling the blindness issue during the interview.

HANDLING THE BLINDNESS ISSUE

Most employers will be afraid to mention your blindness, and will be greatly relieved when you do.

But to manage such a discussion, you must have a firm grasp of the subject yourself. How do you really feel about your blindness? Do you really think it's okay to be blind? If you wish you didn't have to walk with that white cane or dog guide, if you are constantly worried about what people will think when they see you using braille or a magnifying glass, your obvious discomfort will infect those around you.

Becoming comfortable with your blindness is beyond the scope of this book. Suffice to say that getting there is essential to the job-hunting process. Until you realize that alternative work-related techniques—including canes, dogs, readers, drivers, braille, large print, recordings, talking computers, braille printers—enhance your image (because they enhance your productivity), you are not ready to address these important questions in a positive manner during the interview.

Know yourself before you make promises during the interview. If you profess during the interview that you will carry your equal share of the work, but then proceed to do less because of your blindness, you can be sure you will soon find yourself isolated, with little to do.

If you are not willing to work longer hours, hire your own reader, or purchase a piece of equipment, don't say you will. The consequences of trading on your blindness and evading the responsibilities of equal status, while claiming your rights to equal treatment, are far more devastating in the workplace than anywhere else.

Managing a discussion of your blindness is important, but don't allow it to consume the entire interview. With so much to do during the interview, and so little time to do it, you must be prepared to direct the discussion of blindness to *work-related* issues. If an interviewer relentlessly pursues non-job-related topics, such as how you purchase your groceries, "watch" television, fix your meals, etc., it's your job to redirect the conversation back to a discussion of your potential contributions to the organization. You must take control of the interview under these circumstances. Most interviewers will be impressed with your sense of purpose.

On the other hand, if the interviewer resists any effort on your part to seriously discuss the job at hand, chances are you will be looking for work elsewhere.

Think twice, though, about pointing out that such personal questions are probably illegal. Employers are terrified of a potential law suit from a disabled job applicant, which accounts for some of their reluctance to discuss your blindness at all. Very few disabled job seekers get hired after threatening to sue their prospective employers.

OVERCOMING OBJECTIONS AND SELLING YOURSELF DURING THE INTERVIEW

Good salespeople know that every objection raised by a customer is just another chance to sell. The same is true for every job seeker. If you know what objections most employers have about hiring a blind employee, you are in the strategic position of being able to sell yourself during the interview.

Let's look at some of the more common concerns and how you can turn these around to your advantage:

#1 Increased Insurance Rates

Some employers fear that their accident insurance rates would be raised or their insurance carriers would cancel their policies if they hired a blind person. The fear is that blind people are more accident-prone than sighted people. There are no data to support this notion. Besides, group-insurance rates charged to employers are determined by each employer's accident experience and not by the physical characteristics of individual employees covered by the group.

Bring a copy of the leaflet entitled "Insurance Coverage for Blind Workers: Some Facts You Should Know," which is published by the Job Opportunities for the Blind Project for the benefit of employers.

#2 Confidentiality

If you are seeking a job as a counselor or consultant, the employer may express some concern about confidentiality, since your readers would have access to records about clients. Explain that you are personally aware of issues of confidentiality since you, too, must rely on readers to handle your confidential personal mail and checking account. Just as the employer must trust his or her judgment about hiring trustworthy employees to handle confidential records, you also must select readers with integrity.

#3 Why Should I Hire a Blind Worker If I Can Hire a Sighted Worker?

This is the "all other things being equal" argument. But all other things never are equal. We all come into this world and move through it with a mixed bag of strengths and weaknesses.

A person who has no sight may be superior to a sighted peer in intelligence, emotional maturity, manual dexterity, management ability, analytical skill, etc. All job candidates—blind and sighted—should be viewed as *whole* persons. Besides, you may have developed certain qualities as a result of your disability—tenacity, sensitivity, manual dexterity—that make you a stronger candidate than your sighted peers.

#4 But How Can a Blind Person Be a Teacher or a Business Administrator?

Sighted people are dependent on their sight and cannot imagine how they would manage without it. They are convinced that certain tasks require vision, and they cannot conceive of alternative methods which make use of other senses. An employer will not automatically think about the fact that a blind teacher can use a reader to grade papers, or that a business administrator can use a talking computer to calculate budgets.

Even though these alternative techniques are second nature to you, they will have to be spelled out (by you) to unbelieving employers. A hiring manager may think that managers must have sight to do their jobs, when, in fact, the skills of a good manager—understanding people, communicating a vision, motivating staff, defining and solving problems, organizing resources, and devising strategies—are cerebral and interpersonal skills which could be practiced blindfolded.

Even if the job does justifiably require sight, the next question might be, how much sight? Does it require 20/20 vision, or could a legally blind person do the job?

You have already been thinking creatively about how you would do a certain job without sight. You need to communicate this to suspicious employers.

#5 How Will the General Public React to a Blind Employee?

Because most employers are personally uncomfortable with blindness, they fear their customers will be, too. As a result, they tend to hide blind employees in back offices or assign them to jobs with a heavy emphasis on telephone contact or written communication.

There is an analogy here, dating back to the Sixties and Seventies, when blacks and female professionals were relegated to back-room jobs. Today, such practices seem absurd. Employers discovered that the general public could change their attitudes if they were exposed to different kinds of people.

So, if you are offered a telephone customer-service position but would prefer a position dealing with the general public face-to-face, you should state your case. If the employer remains reluctant, you might agree to a starting position dealing with customers on the phone, with the option to move into a position with more direct public contact once you have proved yourself on the job.

#6 Mobility

Since most sighted people envision blindness by closing their eyes, and feeling helpless, they can't imagine blind people traveling comfortably and safely. Your task, again, is to offer information on how, with training and practice, you have come to feel comfortable with your blindness and are able to lead a normal and full life without constantly *thinking* or *worrying* about your lack of sight; about how you travel from here to there, from this city to that, or from this country to another one.

#7 Excessive Absenteeism

This concern stems from the traditional view of blindness as a sickness. As a result, many employers fear that blind workers may be sick more often and consume a disproportionate amount of the organization's health insurance benefits.

There is no evidence to support such fears. In fact, surveys show just the opposite: disabled workers have unusually good attendance records. People—blind or sighted—are individuals. Some will have above-average attendance records, others worse. But it doesn't have anything to do with blindness.

#8 Expense of Adaptive Equipment

Most employers think that job modifications for the blind are very expensive. In some cases, of course, reading machines, computer-access devices, or reader assistance *can* be expensive; but, more often, the accommodations which make a disabled worker productive really are modest.

Often employers operate under the mistaken impression that for a blind employee to be as productive as a sighted one, they must invest in braille elevator panels, steps instead of escalators, regular doors rather than revolving doors, and so on. Your aim during the interview is to explain to the employer the distinction between accommodations that are *necessary* and directly job-related, and accommodations that are *unnecessary* and have little to do with actual job performance.

You should arrange for a third party, such as a rehabilitation agency or service club, to pay for necessary equipment or reader assistance if you cannot afford to do so yourself. But if you can shoulder any of the costs yourself, do so. Your willingness to incur expenses will be viewed by most employers as evidence of your sincere desire to be treated as a contributor. Besides, your task during the interview is to convince prospective employers that they are not taking any more of a risk hiring you than they would in hiring any similarly qualified sighted person. Your job is to reduce the risk factor associated, in the mind of the employer, with your hire.

Once you have the job and have proved yourself as a hard-working and likeable member of the department, you will discover that many employers are more than willing to spend money to increase your productivity and to make your work life more convenient.

Once again, this view of blindness stems from thinking that the loss of sight renders a person helpless. Unfortunately, for some employers this assumption may be supported by actual experience. The interviewer may have personally experienced the burden of employing a blind person who did impose on co-workers, and who did use blindness as an excuse. If you sense that that is the case, you should argue that everyone is an individual, and that people, including blind people, should not be stereotyped because they share one common trait.

Draw on your past work experiences, leisure-time activities, and other examples that show you in a supportive, giving role where others depended on you. Concentrate on the fact that in today's world of work, where the principal focus is on teamwork and cooperation, no one—blind or sighted—is ever wholly independent.

You might discuss briefly how other companies are handling the integration of disabled workers into their labor pools by using a method called job restructuring. Job restructuring is the exchange of tasks between disabled employees and their non-disabled co-workers, in such a way that *all* the members of the department become fully contributing by each making use of his or her strengths. So, for example, in a clerical pool, a totally blind worker may trade copying responsibilities for some of the typing and receptionist duties which originally belonged to a sighted worker.

Successful job restructuring requires imagination and flexibility, both from managers and staff, an ability to view jobs not as fixed sets of tasks, and a willingness to change old work patterns. An IBM manager who was extremely impressed by the speed, accuracy, overall efficiency, and personality traits of a totally blind female applicant made it possible for her to become his full-service secretary simply by modifying some of *his* own old managerial habits. Together they established an office filing system which she could not completely access, but which she could manage sufficiently to suit his needs as long as *he* was willing to provide her with some additional instructions. That way, she was always able to locate and present him with the right document where and when he needed it. The arrangement meant some extra work for him, but it was work which he was prepared to do in order to gain the rare and highly-prized secretarial qualities she offered.

#10 Co-Workers

It's a fact of life that sighted people feel ill at ease in the presence of a blind person. Impress upon the interviewer that you will assume responsibility for making those around you feel more comfortable with your disability. (The interviewer will already have a sense of this from your performance in the interview.)

Remember, though, that your supervisor is the most important person for setting the right tone about your disability. That's one of the reasons it is so important to meet your future boss, face-to-face, as early as possible during the screening process. Avoid letting third parties, such as personnel managers, convey *their* impressions of you, secondhand, to your future boss. You want the chance to evaluate the potential success of your working relationship one-on-one.

#11 Blindness Is Simply Too Restrictive

The overriding but silent concern of most employers is that blind job applicants are simply too restricted to be viable workers. Employers envision blind people working only in limited positions that take advantage of their other senses, such as piano tuner, musician, telemarketer, telephone operator, and so on.

You need to expand the prospective employer's thinking about your capabilities. Offer examples of situations where you made full use of not only your remaining senses of hearing, touch, taste, and smell, but also your native intelligence, for heaven's sake, your imagination, your emotional breadth, and your overall physical agility.

Impress upon your interviewer that you do not live in a "world of darkness," but that you can visualize in your mind's eye not only your immediate environment but the layout of an office building or plant, the geography of a whole city, the map of an entire country, and, for that matter, the globe.

AFTER THE INTERVIEW

Take time after the interview to debrief. Call a trusted friend or counselor and go over the high points (and low points) of the interview. Assess what went well, and think about ways to improve your performance. Do this while the events of the day are still fresh in your mind.

After your emotions have settled, start drafting a letter to the interviewer, thanking him or her for the opportunity to interview for the position. This gives you another chance to mention briefly how your skills and abilities are the perfect match for the job. Show your enthusiasm for the position and for the possibility of working for the prospective employer.

As one seminar participant pointed out:

"The thank-you follow-up note is another opportunity to sell your skills. You can—now that you have more first-hand information about the job—specifically mention how you will perform certain tasks. It's possible that your note will be passed around to folks in other departments to see, in case other people need to be convinced—people who weren't present during the interview."

Then, KEEP WORKING ON YOUR JOB CAMPAIGN. Too many people stop looking for work after one interview, waiting for that call to come which will make them one of the working class—and if it doesn't, feeling devastated and defeated by the process.

Keep the job search alive and active. If you don't stop, it won't be as hard to start up again. Besides, as we said before, the odds are that you will be rejected many times before you are accepted into the fold. It happens that way for everyone.

HERE COMES THE JOB OFFER

Most blind job hunters jump at the first job offer: "I accept!" Who can face the possibility of ongoing rejection when an actual, honest-to-goodness job offer has been made?

At the very least, try to refrain from saying "Yes!" on the spot. Say, instead, "Let me think it over for a few days, if I may." Then sit down and make a list of the pluses and minuses of the job. Try to avoid seeing only the positive aspects. Force yourself to write down the ten best aspects of the job, and the ten worst.

Recognize that a job is more than a title or salary. It means working with a group of people whose personalities may or may not harmonize with yours. It means working with a boss who may or may not see you as a whole person. It means working in a setting which may or may not be compatible with your personal style. Saying "yes" to one job means saying "no" to another, perhaps more suitable, job down the road. It's a big decision affecting every other aspect of your life.

You owe it to yourself to think about it.

Ask yourself, Am I really fascinated by the tasks I will be handling? Will this job make the best use of my skills? Will this position provide me with the right kind of experience at this stage of my career? Is there an opportunity for promotion? If I accept this job, will I be specializing too early in my career? How will this position affect my family?

These questions, and others, should be analyzed carefully before you return that important phone call.

SALARY NEGOTIATIONS

Our purpose in this book is not to duplicate information that can be obtained from other job-hunting guides. We suggest you read several books on salary negotiations; the payoff could be substantial.

But we do offer some advice.

Know what the prevailing salaries are in your field of interest in your part of the country. They will vary considerably from one area to another. Another factor to consider is the salary structure within the particular organization to which you are applying. A small nonprofit agency may pay its managing director less than what a personnel manager makes in a large corporation.

A good resource for salary scales is the U.S. Bureau of Labor Statistics. They conduct and publish the results of area wage surveys, industry wage surveys, and employee benefit surveys, as well as an Annual Survey of Professional, Administrative, Technical, and Clerical Pay. Contact the Bureau's sales office in Chicago.

Professional societies and trade associations often conduct pay surveys among their members and publish the results in their journals and newsletters. Personnel recruitment agencies do the same. Robert Half International, for example, publishes the Annual Survey of Prevailing Financial and Data Processing Starting Salaries.

Stay abreast of what the career columnists and employment-related periodicals are reporting about salary scales. The National Business Employment Weekly regularly reports salary statistics in specific professions.

Make use of your networking contacts, too. Call up someone in the industry and inquire about salary levels. Be careful not to hastily compare your salary offer against the pay rate of someone who may have the same job title but substantially more experience and job responsibilities.

Pay is often dependent on supply and demand. If your skills are in limited supply and high demand, the salary will reflect this situation. If you're not a "hot property," tread lightly. You probably will not be in a position to make non-negotiable demands.

Remember that it's as dangerous to ask for an unrealistic salary as it is to underbid yourself. Why? Because asking for $20,000 when the going rate for the position is $14,000 shows that you are unreasonable, or at least ill-informed. Either way, it doesn't make you look good. Most hiring managers work within a tightly compartmentalized budget. So, while there may be funds to purchase equipment, there may not be more money budgeted for salaries, or vice versa.

When your prospective boss makes you a job offer, ask what the salary range is for the job. Most employers peg the starting salaries of new recruits at or just above the bottom of the pay range, and only in unusual circumstances do they start them above the midpoint of the range. So, in a nonunion setting, you have some room to maneuver. You have less negotiating power in unionized companies or governmental agencies, where the pay system is determined collectively.

If you do press for a higher starting salary, argue your case based on your comparative worth to the employer, and NEVER on your personal requirements "to make ends meet." Employers don't base salaries on individual lifestyles; they pay what the job commands in the marketplace, and according to the level of responsibility. By being informed, you can press for a higher salary based on *facts*, which is impressive to an employer.

In asking for a higher salary, make it clear that you are not turning down the offer. Otherwise, the situation could become a battle of wills, *e.g.,* "If you don't give me the increase, I won't take the job." This is not the way to negotiate. Be more tactful. Say, "It would be easier to accept your offer if the salary was $20-$30 a week higher." Be firm, but pleasant. After all, they have demonstrated that they do want to hire you.

Consider the *entire compensation package* being offered, and not just the weekly salary. For instance, one company might offer you three weeks of vacation instead of two. Or your health-care benefits might be completely covered by one company, and only partially covered by another. One firm might offer an attractive cafeteria-style benefits package, where you can choose between various benefit options. If the health-care plan offers dental insurance, that's money in your pocket. Does the employer offer a tax-deferred annual contribution to a profit-sharing plan?

"Fringes" are no longer fringes, but a very substantial part of the pay package—especially with the escalating costs of health care. At this point, you can ask for a copy of the company's employee benefits handbook. Now that you have a firm job offer, this *is* the time to ask questions about vacations, "perks," and the like.

If your boss will not budge on the salary issue, press for an early review in three or six months. (The norm is 12 months.) Or you may ask for another perk, like tuition reimbursement for a job-related course, or a subscription to a career-related publication.

IT'S NOT OVER YET

You are so happy, so relieved to be rid of the grind of job hunting, that you can't wait to settle down in your new job. No more scanning the newspaper's help-wanted section, no more trips to the library to check out the latest issue of a professional journal in your field, no more monthly meetings of the professional society to which you belong, no more contact with JOB. You have been liberated.

Wrong.

You have convinced one person in one company to give you a chance. Other than that, nothing has changed. All around you, changes in the economy and world of work continue to have an impact on you and your future. The company you joined may be acquired by a larger company next month, leaving you with a boss with whom you can't get along. Or without a job altogether.

So keep your networking contacts *alive*. Drop notes to people and tell them how the job is going. Keep your subscriptions and memberships active. The search for satisfying work isn't over until you celebrate your retirement.

Until then, stay tuned. ¤

Chapter 7
On-the-Job Success
& Upward Mobility

You made it.

You landed the job you worked so hard to get.
Congratulations. But don't sit back in your easy chair yet. It's
time to *prepare* for your first day at work.

First, learn as much as you can about the organization before
you start working. Read the employee handbook, annual
reports, and company newsletters. Second, visit the building
and learn your way around. Bring a sighted assistant along so
you don't disrupt other workers—perhaps even go after-hours.
Third, if possible, get an advance look at the assignments you
will be performing during your first few weeks on the job.

If nothing else, make sure you meet your supervisor and
co-workers before you start working. Imagine this true
scenario: A blind woman was interviewed and hired by a
personnel officer anxious to comply with affirmative action
requirements. The new, blind employee met her surprised
(and shocked) supervisor for the first time when she arrived
for work!

As a blind employee, it may take you a little longer to find your
way around, to arrange for the purchase and installation of
new equipment, and to schedule readers. Therefore, it may
make sense to *volunteer* to come in for a few days, or a week,
to make the necessary arrangements, so that the company is
not paying you for downtime.

But there's another reason for making this extra effort to
insure a smooth start, and that has to do with **image**. If you
arrive for your first day of work and you don't know your way
from the entrance to your desk; if your computer equipment

has not been delivered and hooked up to the company's mainframe; if you don't know who's who, where employees eat lunch, or where the rest rooms are, then the image you project will be one of dependency, lack of productivity, slowness, and inefficiency—an image of, well, not being "on the ball." These are the very same stereotypic impressions that you want to dispel, not reinforce, in the minds of your sighted co-workers and boss.

Another image issue—which should not be ignored—is personal attire. Before you run out and buy a new wardrobe, find out what the unwritten dress code is for *your* position in *that* company. Dress codes range from blue jeans to three-piece business suits; your position within that particular company has its own acceptable standard. If you don't know anyone in the company, call someone in Personnel and inquire about the standard dress code for your position. Explain that you cannot visually assess the dress code, but that you want to comply. Perhaps nothing will do more to improve the first impression others will have of you than the fact that you are suitably attired.

The image you project will be important throughout your tenure with the organization, especially if you aspire to a supervisory position. You want to convey the impression that you are in control of your environment and circumstances, rather than a victim of them. Here are some other steps you should take to project a take-charge image:

¤ If you got your job through the efforts of the rehabilitation agency, limit any direct contact between your counselor and your employer in which you do not take part.

¤ Know where every file or piece of paper is on your desk or in your cabinets, so that you can lay your hands on it quickly whenever your boss or a co-worker asks you for it.

¤ Develop a good memory for names, addresses, telephone numbers, dates, etc., so that you do not have to waste time fishing for a slate and stylus. The ability of many blind people to memorize names, telephone numbers, etc., is always impressive to sighted people, who are notoriously untrained to memorize facts and figures.

¤ Find out where the coffee machine is located and where the photocopying room is. Why? Because these are two areas where people in the organization congregate for informal chitchat. Your ability to get coffee, not only for yourself but also for co-workers, will project an image of self-reliance and, most important, an ability to help others.

One final note of caution: While independence and self-reliance are generally admirable traits, don't let them become a fetish; don't react in a "prickly" manner every time someone offers you assistance, however unnecessary it might be.

MANAGING YOUR BOSS

No relationship is more important than the one with your boss. You should nurture it, cultivate it, and guard it with your life. Not only does your immediate boss have the power to hire, award pay increases, and, within limits, fire those reporting to him or her, but most bosses can also assist subordinates in the advancement of their own careers.

Supervisors vary greatly one from another: Some are excellent "people managers" (that, essentially, is what supervision is all about), others are not; some are highly regarded by their supervisors, others are not. Be patient; don't be overanxious and expect too much too soon.

The following points have been compiled with the better-quality supervisor in mind:

1. Honesty is the best policy in your relationship with your boss. Your openness with him or her regarding your capabilities, weaknesses, and any accommodations you might

require should begin as early as the hiring interview, even before the job offer has been made. Your boss must be able to trust you and rely on your word.

Don't attempt to make any end-runs around your boss. That means, if you cannot persuade your boss to your point of view, don't go directly to your boss's supervisor.

2. At all times, make sure you and your boss have the same expectations of the quantity and quality of the work you are expected to accomplish. Agree with your boss on objectives, results, and procedures at the beginning of each assignment. Don't be afraid to ask questions—even if they seem like dumb ones.

3. Keep the lines of communication open. If you cannot complete an assignment on time, let your boss know immediately. This gives your boss time to make adjustments in his or her plans. At the completion of each major assignment, ask your boss informally for feedback on your work.

4. If company policy requires formal performance appraisals between supervisors and subordinates every 6 to 12 months, you should expect the same consideration. Ask for an evaluation if you don't get one. Don't be content with a "You're doing fine" comment. If you and your boss have been communicating effectively, there should be no surprises during the formal evaluation. Make sure that all conclusions reached during the performance appraisal sessions are put in writing and signed by you and your boss.

5. Perhaps the fundamental reason employers are reluctant to hire blind workers is their assumption that blind employees will necessarily *add* problems, rather than lighten the employers' responsibilities. Work to dispel this prejudicial impression. If you need to go to your boss with a problem—and sometimes you must—be prepared to suggest *solutions* to the problem at the same time.

Understand that your boss, like you, is trying hard to impress his or her superiors. If you work cooperatively with your boss to help make your boss look good, usually your boss will recognize your efforts and reward you accordingly.

6. Ideally, your boss should be willing to advocate on your behalf when others in the organization express skepticism about your abilities and qualifications as a blind employee. You should be careful to not rely exclusively on your boss in this respect. Managers are constantly moving from one position to another; your boss may be there one day, gone the next.

BLINDNESS, PRODUCTIVITY, AND REASONABLE ACCOMMODATION

As we have emphasized many times before, this book is predicated on the philosophy that blind people—with proper training and equal opportunities—can be as productive as their sighted peers. The concept of reasonable accommodation, as defined in the Rehabilitation Act of 1973, as amended, supports this philosophy.

"Accommodation" was never intended to mean a *relaxation* of standards or a *reduction* in the quality and quantity of work expected from the blind employee. Rather, it refers to *variations* in the operating methods and techniques used by blind workers, compared to sighted workers. So, for example, it would be perfectly appropriate for blind medical transcribers to expect the attending physicians to submit their medical reports in recorded form, rather than in writing, as long as the number of typed lines the blind transcribers produced fell within the acceptable standard for all transcribers.

Unfortunately, the correct interpretation of reasonable accommodation has often been misunderstood—by the sighted and the blind alike. Many employers, under pressure from affirmative-action compliance officers, have hired unqualified blind workers simply to fill quotas, while many blind workers have regrettably defined "accommodation" as a *reduction* of the normal job requirements and expectations. The result has damaged the future employability of qualified blind workers.

The finger of blame cannot simply be pointed at the employers or the workers. If qualified blind job seekers are not referred to these employers, and if they are unaware of potential recruitment sources other than the local rehabilitation agency, then these employers have little choice but to hire unqualified blind applicants. At the same time, many blind workers, surrounded by managers and co-workers who consistently expect less of them because of their blindness, slip into the comfortable mindset of expecting less of themselves. They begin to take advantage of their co-workers' natural eagerness to offer excessive and unnecessary assistance. They fail to realize—often until it is too late—what a devastating impact this has on their psyches and on their prospects for career advancement.

If you want to honor the lawful interpretation of reasonable accommodation, consider these strategies:

1. Differentiate between accommodations that are genuinely necessary for you to perform as productively as your sighted co-workers, and those accommodations which would be nice to have but which you could do without.

For example, you may decide that a typewriter would be a necessity, but that a workstation close to the elevator, or braille markings on the elevator, are not really critical. Similarly, you may decide that a computer with accessible output would be a *sine qua non*, but that you could live with a system that is assembled, at relatively little cost, from off-the-shelf components known to the purchasing department, rather than the far more expensive "specially designed" system for the blind user.

Here's a strategy that worked for one seminar participant:

"I think you should be careful about ordering a lot of equipment before you've had a chance to assess the job. I volunteered my time for the first two weeks on the job, during which time I assessed my needs for accommodation. It turned out to be an important time. At first, I didn't think I would need a VersaBraille (a refreshable braille device), but after trying the job for a few weeks, I realized I needed one. But I didn't say to my employer, 'Run out and get me this device.' I went through my local rehabilitation commission and took the major role in getting it on board, including all the frustrations and delays."

As a general rule, you should assume responsibility for figuring out and developing your own accommodations, rather than burdening your employer with another problem. If possible, find out how much various devices cost, and what the company procedures are for ordering new equipment. Obviously, you can't be expected to know everything about adaptive equipment, but you can seek the assistance of people who do.

If your employer *is* interested in being involved in the process, listen constructively to suggestions. Some may be viable, others not, but good managers get paid to synthesize facts to bear on the solution of a problem. You may know how to interface your computer to the company's mainframe, for example, but you may need some interpretative help if the software is graphics-based. Another important consideration, which will involve the company's input, is the desirability of using hardware with which people in the company are familiar, and software which will enable you to share files and other data with others in the department.

2. If you can pay for readers out of your own pocket, or pay for a piece of equipment by taking out a personal loan, offer to do so.

Basically, the company should provide you with any piece of equipment they would normally provide to other co-workers, but asking them to shell out big bucks for the privilege of taking you on board could put you at a disadvantage. Major corporations and government agencies may decline your offer, but smaller organizations with less experience in hiring people with disabilities, and with smaller budgets, will probably find your offer refreshing and indicative of your self-reliant style—and future dedication to the job.

One seminar participant put it this way:

"You have to look at the cost of the piece of equipment in terms of your salary. If it costs three times your salary, what do you expect your employer to say?"

Recognize that once you have proven your worth to the organization, you will be in a better position to request convenience-type accommodations from your employer, and your employer will be much more inclined to make the investment.

3. Through careful observation, identify the "normal" range of productivity among staff members, and measure your own productivity accordingly. It may take a while to get an accurate reading on your co-workers' "normal" output and quality of work—people vary greatly in this area—so don't react negatively if your supervisor claims that your productivity is not up to par. Discuss with your supervisor ways in which you could improve your performance.

Be open to suggestions, even if you think you know the best way to handle a task. One seminar participant shared this story:

"I knew a first-year blind lawyer who had good analytical skills, but found research difficult. The firm was paying for readers, but he insisted on doing research his own way. It took him five times longer than sighted beginning attorneys. The firm's partners tried to help him, but he kept insisting that his research methods were dictated by his blindness and could not be changed.

"Another example involved using a dictaphone. The blind employee insisted on typing his material. The supervisor tried to point out that it's cheaper to have a lower-paid clerk transcribe dictaphone tapes (dictation is 8 times faster than typing), but the employee refused to change his ways.

"The point is, don't be afraid to try new approaches, and remember that you don't have a monopoly on figuring out ways to increase your productivity."

4. Needless to say (we hope), you should never trade on your blindness and impose unnecessary demands on your co-workers. Although you should be alert to negative attitudes toward you as a blind person, be selective about your reactions. Preaching the gospel to a co-worker every time he or she missteps and fails to treat you the same as a sighted person will get tiresome very quickly. As a general rule, good will and constructive discussion always win out over angry confrontation.

SOCIALIZING IN THE WORKPLACE

The personal skills you will need to keep your job and to advance in the organization are quite different from the purely technical skills you need to actually perform the job. Of course, technical skills, knowledge, and competence are important to get the job done. But more important, success in the workplace depends on your *social skills and ability to work with others*. Organizations are made up of people, and people like to do business with people they like. If your social skills are inadequate, if you do not "fit in" well, your co-workers will find ways to work around you. You will begin to feel increasingly isolated and excluded from important company meetings and social events.

Here are some tips for being part of the formal and informal life of the company:

1. Join your co-workers for lunch. If you find you are not being asked, take the initiative. People generally are flattered to be asked to lunch. Do it casually, perhaps even suggesting that you would like to discuss some work-related issue.

2. Participate in after-hours events, like a stop at the local pub. If you are asked at the last moment to join a group at the pub but you have an appointment scheduled with your reader, cancel it. It's more important to go to the pub—even if you don't drink alcoholic beverages. There you will strengthen your social bonds with co-workers and get to know them as people, not just fellow employees.

3. Join the many clubs and interest groups which are often organized in large corporations. At such get-togethers, you will have an opportunity to broaden your circle of acquaintances beyond the co-workers in your own department. Such contacts will be invaluable if you ever want to find out about vacancies, organizational changes, and promotional opportunities in other areas of the organization. Talk to people about their jobs—everyone likes to talk about him- or herself.

4. Organize an occasional party in your own home, and invite both co-workers and personal friends. It's important for your co-workers to see you as a "whole person" with multiple facets, and not only in your 9-to-5 role. Of course, there will always be some co-workers who, for one reason or another—including your blindness—will decline your invitations to lunch or to a party. Don't press them; don't give those around you the impression that you are overeager for their friendship. Just relax and follow what you will come to know as the normal code of social conduct in your particular organization.

5. Be democratic in your socializing: If you happen to be on a professional level, don't limit your socializing to other professionals. Have lunch with secretaries and clerks, too.

(Many secretaries and clerks will keep you plugged in to the organizational grapevine better than anyone else.)

MANAGING PROMOTIONS

The skills you used to get hired are the same skills you will need to get promoted: Preparing resumes, networking, informational interviews, and hiring interviews are all integral parts of the career-advancement process. Let's look at some critical promotion strategies.

As is true in the outside labor market, you need to bring yourself to the attention of potential hiring managers within the organization. Take advantage of opportunities to make formal presentations not only at departmental staff meetings, but also at division-wide and even company-wide gatherings. Volunteer your services on division-wide and company-wide project teams and task forces. Talk to Personnel about possible jobs for which you might qualify in the future, and how you might prepare for them.

If you are in charge of a newsworthy project, look into the possibility of having the editor of the company newspaper write a story about the project, which would include a photograph and pertinent quotations by you. Always look for special assignments which bring you into one-on-one contact with senior executives in the company. Preparing portions of the organization's annual report, making arrangements for a division manager to deliver a speech at the company picnic, or writing the speech for him or her are three examples of high-visibility assignments.

Persuade your boss to register you for company-sponsored training and development programs. You will not only have an opportunity to learn new skills, but you will work closely with a variety of registrants—some of them heads of departments—from different areas of the organization.

MANAGING SUCCESSFULLY
ON THE JOB

In the end, you will succeed on the job, and possibly up the organization, because you have the right skills, the right attitude, and because you really believe you can do it. *You really believe, in your heart of hearts, that you can do it.*

Possibly one of the most damaging forces working against this reality will be other people's lowered expectations, and perhaps some of your own, of your potential contributions to the organization. Work hard to counteract this destructive notion each and every time it presents itself. You are what you believe. Believe in yourself. ¤

Affirmative Action Register
8356 Olive Boulevard
St. Louis, MO 63132
314-991-1335

A Job In Your Future
Dialogue Magazine
3100 Oak Park Avenue
Berwyn, IL 60402
312-749-1908

The American Nurse
American Nurses Association
2420 Pershing Road
Kansas City, MO 64108
816-474-5720

Annual Survey of Prevailing
Financial and Data Processing
Starting Salaries
Robert Half International
111 Pine Street
Suite 1500
San Francisco, CA 94111
415-362-4253

Annual Survey of Professional,
Administrative, Technical and
Clerical Pay
Bureau of Labor Statistics
U.S. Dept. of Labor
230 South Dearborn Street
9th Floor
Chicago, IL 60604
312-353-1880

The Assertive Job Seeker
IN TOUCH NETWORKS
322 West 48th Street
New York, NY 10036
212-586-5588

Atlanta Journal and Constitution
(Sunday Job Guide)
72 Marietta Street NW
Atlanta, GA 30303
800-282-1493 (for subscriptions)
404-526-5151

Audio Cassette Finder
NATIONAL INFORMATION
CENTER FOR EDUCATIONAL
MEDIA
P.O. Box 40130
Albuquerque, NM 87196
505-265-3591

Braille Monitor
National Federation of the Blind
1800 Johnson Street
Baltimore, MD 21230
301-659-9314

Careers and Employment
(see: *Employment and*
Occupations)

CAREERSEARCH (by Jack Erdlen)
The Erdlen Bograd Group, Inc.
20 William Street
Wellesley, MA 02181
617-237-0500

Career World
P.O. Box 3060
Northbrook, IL 60065
312-564-4070

Careers
Elizabeth Fowler
New York Times (Business Day)
229 West 43rd Street
New York, NY 10036
800-631-2500 (for subscriptions)
212-556-1234

321

Careers and the Handicapped
Equal Opportunity
Publications
44 Broadway
Greenlawn, NY 11740
516-261-8899

Chicagoland Job Source
P.O. Box 7125
North Suburban, IL 60199
312-865-7770

Collegiate Career Woman
Equal Opportunity
Publications
44 Broadway
Greenlawn, NY 11740
516-261-8899

Creating Careers with
Confidence
DELTA RAINBOW
98-1020 Kaonohi Street
Aiea, Hawaii 96701
808-488-9873

The Database Directory
Knowledge Industry
Publications
701 Westchester Avenue
White Plains, NY 10604
914-328-9157

Dialogue Magazine
3100 Oak Park Avenue
Berwyn, IL 60402
312-749-1908

Dictionary of Occupational
Titles
Bureau of Labor Statistics
230 South Dearborn Street
9th Floor
Chicago, IL 60604
312-353-1880

Directories in Print
Gale Research
Book Tower
Dept. 77748
Detroit, MI 48277-0748
800-223-4253
313-961-2242

Directory of Executive Recruiters
Kennedy Publications
Templeton Road
Fitzwilliam, NH 03447
603-585-2200

Directory of Internships
National Society for Internship
and Experiential Education
3509 Haworth Drive
Suite 207
Raleigh, NC 27609
919-787-3263

Directory of Online Databases
Cuadra/Elsevier
52 Vanderbilt Avenue
New York, NY 10017
212-916-1150

Directory of Volunteer
Opportunities
Career Resource Center
University of Waterloo
Waterloo, Ontario N2L 3G1
Canada
519-885-1211 ext. 3001

Don't Use a Resume
Richard Lathrop
Ten Speed Press
P.O. Box 7123
Berkeley, CA 94707
800-841-2665
415-845-8414

Employment and Occupations
Superintendent of Documents
U.S. Government Printing
Office
Washington, D.C. 20402-9325
202-783-3238

Encyclopedia of Associations
Gale Research
Book Tower
Dept. 77748
Detroit, MI 48277-0748
800-223-4253
313-961-2242

Federal Jobs Digest
325 Pennsylvania Avenue SE
Washington, DC 20003
800-824-5000
914-762-5111

Forbes Magazine
60 Fifth Avenue
New York, NY 10011
800-772-9200
212-620-2200

From School to Working Life:
Resources and Services
National Library Service for
the Blind and Physically
Handicapped
Library of Congress
Washington, DC 20542
202-707-5100

From Where I Sit
Samuel Feinberg
Women's Wear Daily
7 East 12th Street
New York, NY 10003
212-741-4361

Guide for Occupational
Exploration
AMERICAN GUIDANCE SERVICE
Publishers' Building
Circle Pines, MN 55014
800-328-2560
612-786-4343

(Note: Since the time Chapter
Two was written, the details
regarding the date of publication,
distributor and cost of this
reference work have changed.
The most recently revised edition
of the *Guide* was published in
1984 and is distributed by the
American Guidance Service at a
cost of $34.50. However, as we
reported in Chapter Two, the
unrevised 1979 edition is still
available for $14.00 from the
Superintendent of Documents,
U.S Government Printing
Office.)

Harvard Business Review
Massachusetts Association for
the Blind
200 Ivy Street
Brookline, MA 02146
617-738-5110
800-682-9200 (within
Massachusetts only)

Indianapolis Business Journal
431 North Pennsylvania Street
Indianapolis, IN 46204
317-634-6200

In Search of Excellence
by Tom Peters and Robert
Waterman
Harper and Row Publishers
Keystone Industrial Park
Scranton, PA 18512
800-638-3030
717-824-7300

The Inside Track: How to Get
Into and Succeed In America's
Prestige Companies
by Ross and Kathryn Petras
Random House
400 Hahn Road
Westminster, MD 21157
800-638-6460
301-848-1900

Insurance Coverage for Blind
Workers: Some
Facts You Should Know
JOB OPPORTUNITIES FOR THE
BLIND PROJECT
National Federation of the
Blind
1800 Johnson Street
Baltimore, MD 21230
800-638-7518
301-659-9314

Job Applicant Bulletin
JOB OPPORTUNITIES FOR THE
BLIND PROJECT
National Federation of the
Blind
1800 Johnson Street
Baltimore, MD 21230
800-638-7518
301-659-9314

The Job Seeker's Resource Guide
National Braille Press
88 St. Stephen Street
Boston, MA 02115
617-266-6160

Labor Letter
Wall Street Journal
World Financial Center
200 Liberty Street
New York, NY 10281
800-237-7100 (for subscriptions)
212-416-2000

Lifeprints Close Up
BLINDSKILLS CLOSE UP
P.O. Box 5181
Salem, OR 97304
503-581-4224

Los Angeles Times Index
University Microfilms
300 North Zeeb Road
Ann Arbor, MI 48106
800-521-0600
313-761-4700

Magazines in Special Media
National Library Service for the
Blind and Physically
Handicapped
Library of Congress
Washington, DC 20542
202-707-5100

Manager's Journal
Wall Street Journal
World Financial Center
200 Liberty Street
New York, NY 10281
800-237-7100 (for subscriptions)
212-416-2000

Manhattan, Inc.
P.O. Box 10700
Des Moines, IA 50340
800-777-0444

Marketing Your Abilities
MAINSTREAM, INC.
1030 15th Street NW
Suite 1010
Washington, DC 20005
202-898-0202
202-898-1400

Martindale-Hubbell Law Directory
Martindale-Hubbell, Inc.
630 Central Avenue
New Providence, NJ 07974
201-464-6800

Minority Engineer
Equal Opportunity
Publications
44 Broadway
Greenlawn, NY 11740
516-261-8899

Moody's Industrial Manual
Moody's Investors Service
99 Church Street
New York, NY 10007
800-342-5647
212-553-0300

My Turn
Newsweek
444 Madison Avenue
New York, NY 10022
212-350-4000

National Business Employment Weekly
420 Lexington Avenue
Suite 2040
New York, NY 10170
800-562-4868
212-808-6791

National Newspaper Index
Information Access Company
362 Lakeside Drive
Foster City, CA 94404
800-227-8431
415-378-5000

National Weekly Job Report
Career Link
P.O. Box 11720
Phoenix, AZ 85061
800-331-7717
602-841-2134

Newsletters In Print
Gale Research
Book Tower
Dept. 77748
Detroit, MI 48277-0748
800-223-4253
313-961-2242

Newstrack
P.O. Box 1178
Englewood, CO 80150
800-525-8389
303-778-1692

New York Times Index
University Microfilms
300 North Zeeb Road
Ann Arbor, MI 48106
800-521-0600
313-761-4700

New York Woman
1120 Avenue of the Americas
New York, NY 10036
800-666-5353

Occupational Information Library
Greater Detroit Society for the Blind
16625 Grand River Avenue
Detroit, MI 48227
313-272-3900

Occupational Outlook Handbook
Bureau of Labor Statistics
230 South Dearborn Street
9th Floor
Chicago, IL 60604
312-353-1880

Occupational Outlook Quarterly
Superintendent of Documents
U.S. Government Printing Office
Washington, DC 20402-9325
202-783-3238

The 100 Best Companies to Work for in America
Robert Levering
New American Library
Penquin USA
120 Woodbine Avenue
Bergenfield, NJ 07621
201-387-0600

Online (The Magazine of Online Information Systems)
Online, Inc.
11 Tannery Lane
Weston, CT 06883
203-227-8466

Opportunities in Nonprofit Organizations
ACCESS: NETWORKING IN THE PUBLIC INTEREST
96 Mt. Auburn Street
Cambridge, MA 02138
617-495-2178

The Perfect Resume
by Tom Jackson
Doubleday
P.O. Box 5071
Des Plaines, IL 60017-5071
800-323-9872
312-827-1111

The Personnel Administrator
American Society for Personnel Administration
606 North Washington Street
Alexandria, VA 22314
703-548-3440

Physical Therapy/Occupational Therapy Job News
470 Boston Post Road
Weston, MA 02193
617-899-2702

Rating America's Corporate Conscience
Council on Economic Priorities
30 Irving Place
New York, NY 10003
212-420-1133

Resource Directory of Scientists and Engineers with Disabilities
Project on Science, Technology and Disability
American Association for the Advancement of Science
1333 H Street NW
Washington, DC 20005
202-326-6667

Standard and Poor's Register of Corporations, Directors and Executives
Standard and Poor's
Corporation
25 Broadway
New York, NY 10004
212-208-8787

Standard Periodical Directory
Oxbridge Communications
150 Fifth Avenue
Suite 301
New York, NY 10011
212-741-0231

Summer Employment Directory of the United States
WRITER'S DIGEST BOOKS
1507 Dana Avenue
Cincinnati, OH 45207
513-531-2222

Texas Monthly
P.O. Box 1569
Austin, TX 78767
800-759-2000

Thomas Register (of American Manufacturers)
Thomas Publishing Company
One Pennsylvania Plaza
New York, NY 10119
800-222-7900 ext. 200
212-290-7277

The Three Boxes of Life
Richard N. Bolles
Ten Speed Press
P.O. Box 7123
Berkeley, CA 94707
800-841-2665
415-845-8414

Ulrich's International Periodicals Directory
R.R. Bowker Company
P.O. Box 762
New York, NY 10011
800-521-8110
212-645-9700

Video Source Book
Gale Research
Book Tower
Dept. 77748
Detroit, MI 48277-0748
800-223-4253
313-961-2242

Wall Street Journal Index
University Microfilms
300 North Zeeb Road
Ann Arbor, MI 48106
800-521-0600
313-761-4700

Washington Post
Mail Subscription Department
1150 15th Street NW
Washington, DC 20071
202-334-6000

Washington Post Index
University Microfilms
300 North Zeeb Road
Ann Arbor, MI 48106
800-521-0600
313-761-4700

The Washingtonian
1828 L Street NW
Suite 200
Washington, DC 20036
202-331-0715

What Color Is Your Parachute?
Richard N. Bolles
Ten Speed Press
P.O. Box 7123
Berkeley, CA 94707
800-841-2665
415-845-8414

What's New
New York Times (Sunday
Business)
229 West 43rd Street
New York, NY 10036
800-631-2500 (for
subscriptions),
212-556-1234

*Where Do I Go From Here
with My Life?*
John C. Crystal and Richard
N. Bolles
Ten Speed Press
P.O. Box 7123
Berkeley CA, 94707
800-841-2665
415-845-8414

Who's Hiring Who
Richard Lathrop
Ten Speed Press
P.O. Box 7123
Berkeley, CA 94707
800-841-2665
415-845-8414

Who's News
Wall Street Journal
World Financial Center
200 Liberty Street
New York, NY 10281
800-237-7100 (for
subscriptions),
212-416-2000

*Who's Who in Finance and
Industry*
Marquis Who's Who
3002 Glenview Road
Wilmette, IL 60091
800-621-9669
312-441-2387

The Whole Work Catalogue
New Careers Center
1515 23rd Street
Boulder, CO 80302
303-447-1087

The Working Blind
NATIONAL PUBLIC RADIO
P.O. Box 55416
Madison, WI 53705
800-253-0808
608-263-4892

Working Woman
P.O. Box 10132
Des Moines, IA 50306
800-234-9675

Worklife
PRESIDENT'S COMMITTEE ON
EMPLOYMENT OF PEOPLE WITH
DISABILITIES
1111 20th Street NW
Room 636
Washington, DC 20036
202-653-5044 ¤

ACTION
1100 Vermont Avenue NW
Washington, DC 20525
202-634-9135

ADMINISTRATION ON AGING
(Office of State and Tribal
Programs)
330 Independence Avenue
SW
Washington, DC 20201
202-245-0011

AMERICAN ASSOCIATION OF
RETIRED PERSONS
1909 K Street NW
Washington, DC 20049
202-872-4700

AMERICAN ASSOCIATION OF
UNIVERSITY WOMEN
2401 Virginia Avenue NW
Washington, DC 20037
800-821-4364
202-785-7700

AMERICAN BAR ASSOCIATION
750 North Lake Shore Drive
Chicago, IL 60611
800-621-6159
312-988-5000

AMERICAN CHEMICAL
SOCIETY
1155 16th Street NW
Washington, DC 20036
202-872-4600

AMERICAN COUNCIL OF THE
BLIND
1010 Vermont Avenue NW
Suite 1100
Washington, DC 20005
202-393-3666

AMERICAN MANAGEMENT
ASSOCIATION
135 West 50th Street
New York, NY 10020
212-586-8100

AMERICAN PSYCHOLOGICAL
ASSOCIATION
1200 16th Street NW
Washington, DC 20036
202-955-7600

AREA AGENCIES ON AGING
(see: ADMINISTRATION ON
AGING)

ASSOCIATION OF COLLEGIATE
ENTREPRENEURS
Campus Box 147
Wichita State University
Wichita, KS 67208
316-689-3000

ASSOCIATION OF EXECUTIVE
SEARCH CONSULTANTS
17 Sherwood Place
Greenwich, CT 06830
203-661-6606

ASSOCIATION OF JUNIOR
LEAGUES
660 First Avenue
New York, NY 10016
212-683-1515

ASSOCIATION OF RADIO
READING SERVICES
(Dede Pearse, President)
3124 East Roosevelt Street
Phoenix, AZ 85008
602-231-0500

BETTER BUSINESS BUREAU
(see: COUNCIL OF BETTER
BUSINESS BUREAUS)

BLINDED VETERANS
ASSOCIATION
477 H Street NW
Washington, DC 20001
202-223-3066

BOB ADAMS PUBLISHING, INC.
840 Summer Street
Boston, MA 02127
800-872-5627
617-268-9570

BOSTON COMPUTER SOCIETY
One Center Plaza
Boston, MA 02108
617-367-8080

BRS INFORMATION
TECHNOLOGIES
1200 Route 7
Latham, NY 12110
800-468-0908

BUREAU OF LABOR STATISTICS
U.S Department of Labor
230 South Dearborn Street
9th Floor
Chicago, IL 60604
312-353-1880

BUSINESS AND PROFESSIONAL
WOMEN'S CLUBS
(see: NATIONAL FEDERATION OF
BUSINESS AND PROFESSIONAL
WOMEN'S CLUBS)

CALIFORNIA FOUNDATION ON
EMPLOYMENT AND DISABILITY
(see: FOUNDATION ON
EMPLOYMENT AND DISABILITY)

CAMBRIDGE CAREER PRODUCTS
One Players Club Drive
Charleston, WV 25311
800-468-4227
304-344-8550

CAREER INFORMATION SYSTEM
1787 Agate Street
Eugene, OR 97403
503-686-3872

CAREER PLACEMENT REGISTRY
302 Swann Avenue
Alexandria, VA 22301
800-368-3093
703-683-1085

CAREERTRACK
3085 Center Green Drive
Boulder, CO 80301-5408
800-334-6780 (for seminars)
800-334-1018 (for publications)
303-447-2323

CHRONICLE GUIDANCE
PUBLICATIONS
P.O. Box 1190
Moravia, NY 13118
800-622-7284
315-497-0330

CITIBANK
399 Park Avenue
New York, NY 10022
212-559-1000

COLOZZI, EDWARD A.
DELTA RAINBOW
98-1020 Kaonohi Street
Aiea, Hawaii 96701
808-488-9873

COMPUSERVE INFORMATION
SERVICES
5000 Arlington Center
Boulevard
Columbus, OH 43220
800-848-8199

COUNCIL OF BETTER
BUSINESS BUREAUS
4200 Wilson Boulevard
Suite 800
Arlington, VA 22203
703-276-0100

CSI (Computer Search
International)
Career Network
9515 Deereco Road
Suite 500
Timonium, MD 21093
301-560-0357

CONGRESSIONAL INTERN
PROGRAM
Congressional Intern Office
300 New Jersey Avenue SE
Room 103
Washington, DC 20515
202-226-3621

CONGRESSIONAL PAGE
PROGRAM
(For further information,
contact your U.S. senators or
representative in Congress)

CONTACTS INFLUENTIAL
Trinet, Inc.
9 Campus Drive
Parsippany, NJ 07054
201-267-3600

DAVID TAYLOR RESEARCH
CENTER (Equal Employment
Opportunity Programs)
Code 006
Bethesda, MD 20084-5000
301-227-3359

DELTA GAMMA
3250 Riverside Drive
Columbus, OH 43221
614-481-8169

DEPARTMENT OF LABOR
(see: U.S. DEPARTMENT OF
LABOR)

DIALOG INFORMATION SERVICES
3460 Hillview Avenue
Palo Alto, CA 94304
800-334-2564

DISCOVER
(American College Testing
Program)
230 Schilling Circle
Hunt Valley, MD 21031
301-584-8000

ERDLEN, JOHN (JACK), President
THE ERDLEN BOGRAD GROUP,
INC.
20 William Street
Wellesley, MA 02181
617-237-0500

FOUNDATION ON
EMPLOYMENT AND DISABILITY
3820 Del Amo Boulevard
Suite 304
Torrance, CA 90503
213-214-3430

4-SIGHTS NETWORK FOR THE
VISUALLY IMPAIRED
Greater Detroit Society for
the Blind
16625 Grand River Avenue
Detroit, MI 48227
313-272-3900

FOWLER, ELIZABETH
(see: *Careers* in Publications
List)

THE FOUNDATION CENTER
79 Fifth Avenue
8th Floor
New York, NY 10003
800-424-9836
212-620-4230

FRED PRYOR RESOURCE
CENTER
P.O. Box 2951
Shawnee Mission, KS 66201
800-255-6139
913-384-6400

FUTURE BUSINESS LEADERS
OF AMERICA—PHI BETA
LAMBDA, INC.
P.O. Box 17417—Dulles
Washington, DC 20041
703-860-3334

FUTURE FARMERS OF
AMERICA
(see: NATIONAL FFA
ORGANIZATION)

GALE RESEARCH
Book Tower
Dept. 77748
Detroit, MI 48277-0748
800-223-4253
313-961-2242

HALL, VIRGINIA and WESSEL,
JOYCE
(see: *Atlanta Journal and
Constitution*
SUNDAY JOB GUIDE in
Publications List)

HANDICAPPED ASSISTANCE LOAN
PROGRAM
U.S. Small Business
Administration
1111 18th Street NW
Room 625
Washington, DC 20416
800-368-5855
202-653-6365

INTERNATIONAL ASSOCIATION
OF COUNSELING SERVICES
5999 Stevenson Avenue
Alexandria, VA 22304
800-545-2223
703-823-9800

JIST WORKS
720 North Park Avenue
Indianapolis, IN 46202-3431
800-648-5478
317-637-6643

JOB ACCOMMODATION NETWORK
West Virginia University
809 Allen Hall
P.O. Box 6122
Morgantown, WV 26506
800-526-7234 (out of state)
800-526-4698 or
304-293-7186 (in state)

NATIONAL FEDERATION OF
BUSINESS AND PROFESSIONAL
WOMEN'S CLUBS
2012 Massachusetts Avenue
NW
Washington, DC 20036
202-293-1100

NATIONAL FFA
ORGANIZATION (formerly the
Future Farmers of America)
P.O. Box 15160
Alexandria, VA 22309
703-360-3600

NATIONAL LIBRARY SERVICE
FOR THE BLIND AND
PHYSICALLY HANDICAPPED
Library of Congress
Washington, DC 20542
202-707-5100

NATIONAL PUERTO RICAN
FORUM
31 East 32nd Street
New York, NY 10016
212-685-2311

NATIONAL TECHNOLOGY
CENTER
American Foundation for the
Blind
15 West 16th Street
New York, NY 10011
212-620-2079

NEWSNET
945 Haverford Road
Bryn Mawr, PA 19010
800-345-1301
215-527-8030

NEW YORK CITY DEPARTMENT
FOR THE AGING
2 Lafayette Street
15th Floor
New York, NY 10017
212-577-8441

NIGHTINGALE-CONANT
CORPORATION
7300 North Lehigh Avenue
Chicago, IL 60648
800-323-5552
312-647-0300

ONLINE CHRONICLE
Online, Inc.
11 Tannery Lane
Weston, CT 06883
203-227-8466

OREGON COMMISSION FOR THE
BLIND
535 SE 12th Street
Portland, OR 97214
503-238-8375

PEACE CORPS
1990 K Street NW
Washington, DC 20526
800-424-8580

PRESIDENT'S COMMISSION ON
WHITE HOUSE FELLOWSHIPS
712 Jackson Place NW
Washington, DC 20503
202-395-4522

PRESIDENT'S COMMITTEE ON
EMPLOYMENT OF PEOPLE WITH
DISABILITIES
1111 20th Street NW
Room 636
Washington, DC 20036
202-653-5044

PROJECT JOB SITE
New York Association for the
Blind
The Lighthouse
111 East 59th Street
New York, NY 10022
212-355-2200

PROJECT ON SCIENCE,
TECHNOLOGY AND DISABILITY
American Association for the
Advancement of Science
1333 H Street NW
Washington, DC 20005
202-326-6667

PROJECT WITH INDUSTRY
Rehabilitation Services
Administration
U.S. Department of
Education
Switzer Building
Room 3320
330 C Street SW
Washington, DC 20201
202-732-1333

RABBY, RAMI
136 E. 55th Street
Suite 8E
New York, NY 10022
212-371-7766

RADIO READING SERVICE
(see: ASSOCIATION OF RADIO
READING SERVICES)

RECORDED PERIODICALS
Associated Services for the
Blind
919 Walnut Street
Philadelphia, PA 19107
215-627-0600

ROBINSON, PEGGY (Area
Manager)
MANPOWER, INC.
99 Summer Street
Suite 1520
Boston, MA 02110
617-439-4321

ROTARY INTERNATIONAL
1 Rotary Center
1560 Sherman Avenue
Evanston, IL 60201
312-866-3000

SECURITIES INDUSTRY
ASSOCIATION
120 Broadway
35th Floor
New York, NY 10271
212-608-1500

SIGI +
P.O. Box 6403
Princeton, NJ 08541
800-524-0491
215-750-8110

THE SOURCE
1616 Anderson Road
McLean, VA 22102
800-336-3366
703-734-7500

SUPERINTENDENT OF
DOCUMENTS
U.S. Government Printing Office
Washington, DC 20402-9325
202-783-3238

SURREY BOOKS
101 East Erie Street
Suite 900
Chicago, IL 60611
312-751-7330

TELEPHONE PIONEERS OF
AMERICA
22 Cortlandt Street
Room C2575
New York, NY 10007
212-393-6288

TEN SPEED PRESS
P.O. Box 7123
Berkeley, CA 94707
800-841-2665
415-845-8414

U.S. BUREAU OF LABOR
STATISTICS
(see: BUREAU OF LABOR
STATISTICS)

U.S. DEPARTMENT OF LABOR
200 Constitution Avenue NW
Washington, DC 20210-0001
202-523-6666

U.S. EMPLOYMENT
OPPORTUNITIES
Washington Research
Associates
P.O. Box 32096
Washington, DC 20007
703-276-8260

VERSABRAILLE USERS GROUP
c/o David Goldstein, Editor
VersaNews
87 Sanford Lane
Stamford, CT 06905
203-336-4330 (home)
203-366-3300 (work)

WOMEN IN COMMUNICATIONS
2101 Wilson Boulevard
Suite 417
Arlington, VA 22201
703-528-4200

WOMEN IN MANAGEMENT
2 North Riverside Plaza
Suite 2400
Chicago, IL 60606
312-263-3636

YMCA of the USA NATIONAL
HEADQUARTERS
101 North Wacker Drive
14th Floor
Chicago, IL 60606
800-872-9622
312-977-0031

YOUNG AMERICANS BANK
250 Steele Street
Denver, CO 80206
303-321-2265

YWCA of the USA NATIONAL
BOARD
726 Broadway
5th Floor
New York, NY 10003
212-614-2700 ¤